Dancing Away an Anxious Mind

Dancing Away an Anxious Mind

A Memoir about Overcoming Panic Disorder

Robert Rand

THE UNIVERSITY OF WISCONSIN PRESS
TERRACE BOOKS

The University of Wisconsin Press
1930 Monroe Street
Madison, Wisconsin 53711

www.wisc.edu/wisconsinpress/

3 Henrietta Street
London WC2E 8LU, England

1   3   5   4   2

Printed in the United States of America

Library of Congress Cataloging-in-Publication Data
Rand, Robert.
Dancing away an anxious mind: a memoir about overcoming panic disorder /
Robert Rand.
p.   cm.
ISBN 0-299-20164-3 (cloth: alk. paper)
1. Rand, Robert.
2. Dancers—United States—Psychology—Anecdotes.
3. Folk dancing, Cajun—United States—Psychological aspects—Anecdotes.
I. Title.
GV1588.5.R36   2004
792.9′092—dc22   2004005368

Terrace Books, a division of the University of Wisconsin Press,
takes its name from the Memorial Union Terrace, located at
the University of Wisconsin–Madison. Since its inception in 1907,
the Wisconsin Union has provided a venue for students, faculty, staff,
and alumni to debate art, music, politics, and the issues of the day.
It is a place where theater, music, drama, dance, outdoor activities, and
major speakers are made available to the campus and the community.
To learn more about the Union, visit www.union.wisc.edu.

For ERIKO

Contents

I
Tornado Alley

The great outposts of civilization are often distinguished by pillars and gold, by magnificent flying buttresses that arch beneath cathedral domes, by cement and steel temple mounts that rise from city sidewalks to scrape against the clouds. But sometimes they're signaled by simpler things. At Tornado Alley, near Washington, D.C., civilization meant music and dance, marked with a side of barbecue.

Roadhouse, juke joint, urban ballroom. Tornado Alley was all that: a delicious soup of live bands and rhythm and blues; of amplified riffs on a squeeze box or guitar that hissed and sizzled like steaks on a griddle, drawing patrons to a dance floor that was frayed from overuse; of pulled pork and collard greens served with corn bread and slaw on polystyrene plates with plastic knives and forks.

"The hickory-smoked chicken is stunning," the *Washington Post* once reported. "The ribs are similarly flavorful, meaty, and easy off the bone."

At Tornado Alley, diners sat in straight-backed wooden booths that looked like church pews and bruised the posterior. The act of eating was difficult. The kitchen deferred to the dance floor.

The club had a noteworthy history. It was the reincarnation of Twist and Shout, the famous but defunct dance joint that Washington-based singer-songwriter Mary Chapin Carpenter memorialized in a Grammy Award–winning song.

"Saturday night and the moon is out, I wanna head on over to the Twist and Shout," Carpenter wrote. "Find a two-step partner and a Cajun beat, when it lifts me up I'm gonna find my feet. Out in the middle of a big dance floor, when I hear that fiddle wanna beg for more. Wanna dance to a band from Louisian' tonight."

Louisiana music was the signature sound at the old Twist and Shout. The tradition survived the club and now prospered at Tornado Alley.

A man in a T-shirt and jeans arrived at the club one November evening at ten o'clock. He was early middle-aged. A pair of leather dance shoes covered his feet. The soles were scored and scratched. They had been to Tornado Alley before.

He walked through the doors of the canopied entrance and paid an eight-dollar cover charge. Once inside, a wall of accordion music cut him short, compelling his attention.

"Eh toi! We're doin' zydeco in the house t'night, y'all!"

To his left, on a platform stage at the edge of a packed parquet dance floor, stood a locomotive of a man: head back, shoulders erect, eyes forward. He towered above the crowd, pumping and plying his button accordion with the artistry and focus of a sculptor kneading clay.

The sound that emerged was arresting: a reedy, percussive tremolo of driving treble riffs and booming bass chords that lumbered down the tracks and overtook the hall.

> CHANK-a-chank-a-CHANK-a-chank-a,
> CHANK-a-chank-a-CHANK-a-chank-a.
> CHANK-a-chank-a-CHANK-a-chank-a,
> CHANK-a-chank-a-CHANK-a-chank-a.
> *Okay, we're rollin', baby. Have mercy! Ooo-eeee!*

Roy Carrier, the man onstage, screwed up his eyes and looked to the heavens and smiled a slight, knowing smile, as if God himself had shucked his tie and set about to zydeco. Zydeco and Cajun music are first cousins, with roots in the prairies of French-speaking South Louisiana, in back-country towns with lyrical names like Lawtell and Eunice, Opelousas and Mamou. The zydeco and Cajun sounds, on the surface, are similar, primed with the sonorous, pleasing call of the accordion. But Cajuns are white, and so is their music. Zydeco came from a different place, from Louisiana's black Creole culture. These were rural African Americans, a people once so impoverished that many lacked the funds to buy a trace of salted meat to season up their snap beans. *"Les haricots sont pas salés"*—"the snap beans aren't salty"—they used to say. "Les haricots" is pronounced "lay ZAH-ree-coe." Zydeco. That's the derivation of the music's name.

Roy Carrier was as fine a proselytizer of zydeco as ever there was. He had the dignity and presence of a man his age, which was fifty-some years. But he was hip, too, in an understated sort of way, with a black leather cap and greased-down curls and a fuzzy goatee that made his music young. Then there were his hands: big, fleshy, oil-worker hands with meaty fingers—the tip of one was missing—that overwhelmed the squeeze box he cradled on his chest.

> CHANK-a-chank-a-CHANK-a-chank-a,
> CHANK-a-chank-a-CHANK-a-chank-a.
> CHANK-a-chank-a-CHANK-a-chank-a,
> CHANK-a-chank-a-CHANK-a-chank-a.
> *We're havin' a good time over in the house*
>   *tonight, y'all. Yeah, you right!*

Surrounding Roy were the Night Rockers—a drummer, lead guitarist, bass guitarist, and rubboard player. The metal rubboard, or frottoir, is zydeco's trademark instrument. Resembling a corrugated stainless-steel vest that is harnessed to the shoulders, the frottoir gives the music backbone, and grounds it with energy and sparkle.

The Night Rockers' rubboardist was eighteen years old and beanstalk thin. But his frottoir provided bulk and power. He attacked the instrument with jackhammer zeal, whipping his arms up and down as they beat a pair of metal strikers across the rubboard's jagged face. The instrument's voice was flat and coarse, like sandpaper on metal. But the rubboardist knew how to nail a rhythm, with repetitive phrases that mesmerized and drove the music forward.

> CHICK-u-tuh CHICK-u-tuh CHICK-u-tuh CHICK-u-tuh
> CHICK-u-tuh CHICK-u-tuh CHICK-u-tuh CHICK-u-tuh,
> CHANK-a-chank-a-CHANK-a-chank-a,

CHANK-a-chank-a-CHANK-a-chank-a,
Diggy diggy DUM, diggy diggy DA, some-body
TELL me, that's ZYDECO!
Diggy diggy DUM, diggy diggy DA, some-body
TELL me, I wanna ZYDECO!

Roy's voice was also flat and coarse, and the lyrics he sang were sparse, and deliberately so, for this was dance music, and the marriage of the voice, frottoir, and accordion had but one purpose: to stir passions, to get people up and moving.

"If you hear the zydeco, and you don't move, then you dead." That's what they say about zydeco down in South Louisiana. Listen to it, just for an eight-count, and Lord help you if some extremity of your anatomy doesn't start to twitch or quake.

There were five hundred square feet of wood parquet floor in Tornado Alley, and all of it had filled by the time the man in the T-shirt and jeans had entered the club. Some forty pairs of dancers surged and pulsed before him. They moved intently, with introspective smiles, as if carried away in a trance by the repetitious mantra of the zydeco beat. Some were athletic and fit. Some were overweight. Some of the men wore ponytails. So did some of the women. Nearly all of the people were white, and most had exited their twenties.

The faces he saw were familiar. A curly-gray-haired government lawyer with a bandanna in his hand and a Panama hat atop his head, which he'd tip to his partner at the end of each dance. A medical doctor, in sexy black hose and a red miniskirt, with a red carnation in her hair. A delivery driver, the most regal dancer of all, in a long-sleeved shirt, white Levi's, and a posture that earned him respect. The raven-haired environmentalist, with an airy blouse, white ankle socks, and slacks that hugged and offered up a most appealing figure.

A Federal Reserve economist was on the dance floor. A pollution fighter from the EPA. A nurse. An architect. A therapist. A scientist. A White House political appointee. Chameleons who shed their daytime colors and became something else when they visited Tornado Alley.

The music stopped for a moment, and Roy Carrier mopped the sweat from his forehead, catching his breath before the next song. Most of the dancers remained on the dance floor, shuffling around and shifting partners as if they were playing musical chairs. In this version of the game, however, the competition ended when the music started up, and the losers, not the winners, were the ones who got the chairs, forced to sit partnerless on the sidelines, unable to join the next round of dance.

The man in the T-shirt and jeans stepped into the mix in search of a partner of his own. He wanted a woman who knew what she was doing. That was the best way to zydeco.

He found Coco planted near the foot of the stage.

"Well, hiiiii!" she squealed, as he approached. "So nice to see you here!"

"Hi there, Coco," he said.

Coco, a teacher in her middle thirties with an ever pleasant disposition, wrapped her arms around his waist with a welcoming hug. The gesture made him feel good, for he was quite fond of her.

"You free to dance?" he asked.

"You betcha," Coco said.

They joined in the closed position, the well-established ballroom stance. He took her right hand with his left, and drew it gently outward. The grip they'd formed was strong and certain, for they had done this many times before. Coco had been his dance instructor, the woman who helped him to find his dance-floor feet.

His right arm reached around her waist, where his palm settled low upon her back, to support and to guide her movements. Her left arm rose and found a spot to rest on his right shoulder. It was all familiar ground. The space between them closed a bit, as they readied for the music.

"Eh toi, baby! Fais 'tention, baby! We're havin' a party tonight, I guar-own-tee!"

Roy Carrier bore down on the bellows of his squeeze box, and a swell of sound, fat with energy and spirit, rolled out from the stage. Coco drew a breath and tightened the grip on her partner's shoulder. He squeezed her palm and flexed his knees. And the two of them exploded.

> *Step-pause-quick-quick, step-pause-quick-quick.*
> *Left-right-right-left, right-left-left-right.*

Steppausequickquick, steppausequickquick.
Leftrightrightleftrightleftileftright.

Faster and faster they went, first left and right, then right and left, then round and round in a four-legged whirlwind. Their arms strained to contain the centrifugal force of their common enterprise. The space between them closed even more, and soon their thighs had interlocked, not for any prurient interest, but simply because the movement was stabler that way.

Within the blur, they looked at each other, square in the eye, as they twisted and turned to the music. Their gaze held, anchoring the dance.

Suddenly, unexpectedly, he whooped with glee.

Coco laughed. So did he. And the smiles they shared were unconstrained, like the purr of a kitten, defining the joy of the moment.

The man on that dance floor was me, and I remember thinking back then, amidst the rush of the experience, that I had somehow—finally—pummeled my life into a happy state of submitting to unbridled pleasure. That the process involved social dance was all the more stunning, for I was a serious, temperate man whose instincts, throughout my life, had led me to cower at public displays of frolic. It was an unhealthy mind-set—pathologically so—that eventually triggered a full-blown psychiatric crisis that crippled my spirit and threatened my health for way too many years.

Coco had taught me just how much fun dancing could be, and fun was the serum I sorely needed to heal and to grow. But changing who you are, altering well-established patterns of thought and behavior, discarding the cycle of acts and omissions that gave you your problem in the first place—these are exacting things. It is easier to suffer. So my passage to the dance floor, and to recovery, was not direct, and certainly not easy.

2
Dancing and Me

I was a nondancer for most of my life, raised in a household where propriety, self-control, and dignity were served with mashed potatoes for dinner. Well mannered. Pensive. Scholarly. Serious. I was all that. A good boy. A very good boy. The perfect son, programmed by perfect parents to be a perfectionist.

As such, random and aberrant gesticulation of body parts was not encouraged. The Rands did not twist, shake, rattle, or roll. Not in private. And certainly not in a public forum. Imagine, as I did back then, the mortification I would bring unto myself and my loved ones should I ever attempt to move to a song. It just wouldn't happen. I was too shy. Too self-conscious. Too fearful of what others might think. Boogie was not in my gene pool.

Music, however, in its unadulterated form, was okay. It was even fostered, as long as it stayed at the piano. The piano was my childhood ballroom. My fingers could dance there, up and down the octaves, and my body could even sway on its perch at the bench, for at the piano, the movements were genteel, scripted by Mozart or Bach: perfect little sonatinas, performed to a T by the well-tempered student.

My uncle Ted never played the piano. He did like to dance, though. And so did my aunt Gert. At a wedding or bar mitzvah they'd take to the dance floor, and fueled by a pair of high-octane smiles they'd flail their arms and fling their legs and twirl in tight little circles that stirred up convention and embarrassed their relations.

Uncle Ted and Aunt Gert had fun. Significant fun. And as such they were suspect.

I remember the first time I tried to dance. It was New Year's Eve. The early sixties. I was eight or nine years old, and our clan had gathered at Ted and Gert's house to celebrate. We played Monopoly and poker and ate pizza and carry-out chicken with Vernor's ginger ale.

After midnight, Uncle Ted dragged me and my sister and my two cousins out to the living room carpet and lined us up execution-style in front of a turntable and a couple of speakers. It was time to cha-cha, he declared.

He put on some record—Stan Getz, I think—and he started to speak in tongues: One, two, cha cha cha. Three, four, cha cha cha. And he told us to move our feet to a cha-cha beat: left, right, left-right-left; forward, back, step-in-place. And, being good kids, we did as we were told. I remember my cousins delighting in the experience, while I stood there, timid and paralyzed. At some point Uncle Ted grabbed my hands and in front of everybody attempted to lead me through the cha-cha pattern.

"Attaboy, Robby, you can do it," he said. "One, two, cha cha cha. Left, right, left-right-left."

I blushed and bungled the whole thing. I was traumatized and imperfect. It was going to be a bad year.

During the next decade, social and political upheaval stirred the country. So did rock and roll. I watched it all on *American Bandstand.* Dance forms injurious to the nation's well-being. Dance forms designed to riot and ruin. Dance forms that I would never have the temerity to do: The pony. The monkey. The Watusi. Outrageous, uncontrolled gyrations by America's misguided youth.

Each Saturday I'd sit in my bedroom and observe the spectacle with the door closed, so as not to alarm my parents. I'd stare at the TV with a mixture of sheepish fascination and scorn as my peers shook their behinds with bravado and—I had to acknowledge—enviable abandon. They wore hippie hairdos and had psychedelic eyes. They also wore Ted and Gert's smiles. No matter. Their behavior was inappropriate. Embarrassing. "I'm glad I'm not like them," I'd tell myself.

By the time I reached eighteen, my attitude toward dancing was pretty much set. It was simply something I would not and could not do. Until Karla Rosenzweig and the senior prom came along.

Karla was my first love. My high school sweetheart. She was drop-dead gorgeous, with long brown hair and genuine female curves that seriously threatened my virginity. She was also as outgoing and filled with self-assurance as I was awkward and introspective. She was a singer and actress. I read Dostoyevsky. I was socially timid. She was wonderfully unabashed. Karla had what I didn't, and I wanted what she had.

Karla, like most free spirits, liked to dance. So when senior prom came around, after the celebratory dinner at some fancy country club, I found myself straddling the edge of a ballroom dance floor, a tuxedo-wrapped jumble of anxiety, forced by the love of a woman to walk the plank.

There was no way I could get out of it. The stakes were too high; the shame of demurral and of letting Karla down was greater than the embarrassment I'd suffer from attempting to dance.

It was 1971, and dance music—if you were eighteen, white, middle class, and suburban—was an odd mix of steel and maple syrup. The Rolling Stones, the Doors, and other cutting-edge ensembles provided the hard stuff, the music with electric underbelly and machine-gun rhythms; the sweetness came from groups like the Archies (their hit tune was called "Sugar, Sugar") and the McCoys ("Hang on, Sloopy")—lollypop rock for people who liked to play it safe. It was all, however, music of that era, music that demanded attention, and music—alas, at a high school prom—that required movement. Even when Manny Dermer and his orches-tra performed it.

It goes without saying that I went to the prom un-equipped. I would not be able to perform on the dance floor with the kind of poise and perfection the world expected of me, or I expected of myself. In a gracious humanitarian gesture, Karla had arranged a couple of predance practice sessions in the basement rec room of her parents' house. She tried to teach me the box step. A lot of good that would do to "In-A-Gadda-Da-Vida."

In fact, there were two and only two dance forms that teenagers in my part of the world did back then: freestyle, where a young man and young woman faced each other three feet apart and, never touching, jiggled herky-jerky every which way to the music; and slow dancing, a hormonally driven exercise, in which a couple embraced so the guy could feel full force the weight and allure of the girl's bosom, and the girl could feel the bump in the front of his pants, and, if she chose, could adoringly rest her head on his shoulder as they swayed back and forth, like a metronome, until death, or graduation, did them part.

We did both forms of dance that evening, Karla and I. I distinctly remember two separate forays. The first was most painful—a callous set of fast instrumentals to which I box-stepped rather stiffly all by myself: first left, then forward, then right, then back, over and over and over again no matter the song, my arms all the while hanging down by my sides like a couple of noodles, deaf to the music, while Karla, God bless her, pranced joyfully before me, my dancing angel, her beauty and undulating body enough to spur me on.

The second set, more forgiving, involved slow dancing, and that I could handle, for handling Karla was no great chore, and riding the waves of her lilting torso was any boy's dream. We danced to the Carpenters' classic "We've Only Just Begun": me in a blue tux with blue velvet piping, mile-wide collars, velveteen bow tie, and a powder-blue shirt with ruffles; she in a light-blue chiffon dress with an empire waist and a lace bodice. "We were," Karla said, "entirely too cute for words."

At the end of the evening I blinked and I sighed and I realized, albeit briefly, that I had enjoyed myself. And I pledged that it would never, ever happen again.

It certainly didn't in college, which I finished in three years with straight As, two majors, highest honors, and the social life of a recluse. I lived at home with my parents, commuting to classes five days a week. A Saturday night meant a six-pack of donuts and Hegel or Nietzsche. You can't dance to either of them.

I didn't have fun in graduate school, either, though in graduate school I did for a time join a folk-dancing cult.

Folk dancing, to me at least, was not really dancing, and not really fun. It was, instead, interesting: a moral academic imperative, part of my major in Slavic studies, and justifiable, therefore, under the circumstances.

I was drawn in particular to the Bulgarian line dance, and for a time I made it my own. It was quite the scene: guys dancing with guys, yelping and sweating to the quick-quick-slow rhythm of the *ruchenitsa,* a traditional genre of folk tune. The experience was, to be honest, quite mesmerizing, as the drone of the *gaida,* a Bulgarian bagpipe, lured us snakelike through the line of movement, one stomping leg at a time. It was macho, like football. And it also was scholarly: intricate Balkan harmonies yearning to flee the Communist yoke, exotic Cyrillic steps that were simple and predictable and could be studied and mastered and even researched in the library. No improvisation or spontaneity was required here. There was no shame before parents, nor public embarrassment. This was serious dancing. Dance without smiles. The perfect art form.

I gave it up when I left graduate school.

Another ten years would pass before I took to the dance floor again. It was 1983. Reagan was president. Disco was dying. America had finally come to its senses.

A new woman had entered my life. A woman I wanted to marry. Her name was Jeanette. She was as beautiful and free-spirited and kindhearted as Karla. And—God is cruel—twice the dancer.

I managed, for the most part with Jeanette, to avoid situations where dancing might transpire. I lured her, quite by design—and, I might add, with considerable guile and charm—to venues where movement and music did not coexist. Hiking. Running. Biking. Films. Dance-free activities all. Safe havens. She didn't even know what she was missing.

At the occasional house party we attended, however, when the music went on and the outbreak of dancing seemed imminent, I'd gather my legs and repair to the kitchen, stealthily, like a combat deserter. There I'd hide—perhaps *cower* is a better word—to engage some other nondancing guest in serious conversation about Kremlin politics or antiballistic-missile systems.

Once, when I peered out of my kitchen sanctuary, I saw that Jeanette had begun to dance in the other room. All by herself. Rocking to and fro to the Rolling Stones. Churning her arms and wiggling her hips in an understated but most appealing manner as a circle of onlookers applauded.

I pretended not to notice. But I did, of course. And I was ashamed, because I was Jeanette's boyfriend and I should have been out there dancing by her side. And I was angry, because Jeanette knew I hated to dance, yet she stepped out and danced without me, drawing attention to my absence and to the cowardice it represented. And I was jealous, jealous of how good she looked and how well she danced and how inadequate and imperfect that made me feel. And I saw how the other guys eyed her. And I resented the way they watched her every move, the way they craved her pulsating loins. I felt like a cuckold.

I remembered that feeling, some months later, when Jeanette and I attended a wedding. I was in night law school at the time, and my classmate and friend Randi was marrying a man named Myles, who had clerked at the U.S. Supreme Court. It was a big, elegant affair. Hundreds of people were there. Guests had their choice of beef or chicken or fish. A video-production team was hired to record the event. And there was dancing, and lots of it.

The band was Lou Ginsberg's. The music was Jewish American corn pone, light-rock Hava Nagilah. We passed on the horas. But when Lou started in on the rock-and-roll standards, by Elvis and Mick and Tina and Elton, I looked at Jeanette, who was all dolled up, and she looked at me with her puckish green eyes, and I was a goner.

"You wanna dance?" I asked.

She nodded, and within seconds we were on the dance floor.

It was shame, for the most part, that drew me there. I was ashamed to let her down, as I had at the party. Ashamed to have her sit there, all coiled up and ready to spring, held back by my fears. Ashamed at the prospect of some other guy asking her to dance, and of her saying yes. Ashamed at the prospect of having to explain, on the ride home, why I'd ruined the evening, why I wouldn't dance.

So dance I did.

My tactics were straightforward, if not particularly clever: since I didn't know how to dance, I'd copy and mimic Jeanette, who did. She would slither on the dance floor in that wonderfully fluid way of hers, a few steps forward, a few back, her hips jutting oh so subtly left and then right. She'd punctuate every beat with a jut of the arm or a jog of the head and a hint of sensuality that made her dangerous and dignified, all at the same time. And I would follow, literally walking in her wake, plodding the best I could, a mirror image of my lady, advancing and retreating to the strains of the music: one-two, one-two, hitting the floor with my feet, my torso maneuvering here and there, deployed, for better or worse, in a posture of no retreat.

And after a while I remember snapping my fingers just as Jeanette did—snap-pause, snap-pause—to the cadence of a tune, and I surprised myself in doing so, for I was moving my legs at the time. And Jeanette was smiling. And so was I. And it felt really good. Really good. And it was a moment I wouldn't repeat for another five years, for I was a serious fellow, with serious work to do, and dancing was not in my blood. Yet it was also a moment I'd never forget: a hint of what could be, a seed that would lie dormant, deep inside me, until years later, when desperation intervened and cracked open its husk, releasing the stuff that would nurture me back to health.

"I'd say it was something about wanting to do everything well and fearing you'd do something badly, and in public yet." That's how Jeanette explained my fear of dance. Dancing, she said, would have been "a useful exercise in not taking yourself too seriously." She was right, of course. If only I had taken her counsel and eased up a bit. That's what I needed to do. Stop striving for perfection in each and every aspect of my life. Have some fun, for God's sake. Dance.

One month after Jeanette and I broke up, I visited

Chicago, my hometown, and met with a couple of old high school friends. Van and Iris knew me before Jeanette, and even before Karla. They were real pals, always there no matter what. Their comfort was just what I needed to help me forget a broken relationship, and a broken heart.

It was the Fourth of July, and the three of us made a day of it. We picnicked and watched the fireworks and strolled arm in arm along the lakefront. We talked about all kinds of things, old teachers, old hijinks, old flames. And after the fireworks had ended, we walked down to Lincoln Avenue and went to a club to hear music.

It was dance music. Rock and roll. Van and Iris jumped the boogie. I just stood there, self-conscious, embarrassed, immobilized. All the old feelings.

Later on, after Van had left, Iris took my hand, fixed on my eyes, and looked inside me.

"Don't you ever cut loose, Robby?" she asked. "You know, just cut loose?"

She posed the question tenderly enough, moved not by malice but by friendship and instinct that told her something was not quite right.

I stared at her, though, angered by the directness of her question, which spoke the truth.

I told her I didn't want to talk about it. She said okay.

We went back to her apartment and had sex instead.

I shall not reveal here and now the complete nature of what finally and irrevocably pushed me onto the dance floor. Better to meet the disease as I did: unwittingly, over time.

It first came calling in 1988, two and a half years after Jeanette and I had parted ways. I had fled to Russia on a fellowship, to Moscow, to research a book and to forget Jeanette, whose memory lingered on. My work in the Soviet capital was serious and intense. I had quit a job to go there. My future depended on the success of my project, and I was determined, as always, not to fail. There were very long hours of reporting and research. The living conditions were difficult. Long lines for food. A shortage of everything. Inadequate heat. Obdurate bureaucrats. Life in Moscow just chipped away at you, day after day after day.

I was in a theater one afternoon with a female friend when my psychiatric affliction first appeared. It came on suddenly, out of nowhere, from within. It shook me hard, like a bully, and it dumped me on my knees, dizzy and beaten up. I could barely breathe.

"Izvinitye, mnye plokho," I said to my friend. "Excuse me, I'm not well."

I left the theater to take in some fresh air. The bad feelings eventually passed.

I dismissed the experience as a virus, or perhaps the effect of some spoiled food I had eaten. When it happened again, again at the theater, I figured it must be an allergy, for Russian women wore potent perfumes when out on the town, and their scents, I guessed, for me could be noxious. One fragrance in particular, *Krasnaya Moskva*—Red Moscow—was an especially popular and sickeningly pungent concoction.

So I avoided the playhouse, and the cinema, too. And I felt certain that what I had suffered was nothing to be concerned about.

But my mood turned increasingly dour, and my strength diminished. An angry Moscow winter melted into an inhospitably muddy spring. The skies were Russian gray. My workload refused to lighten. I was to leave Russia soon, and there was still much to do.

I passed one week in April alone, in my room, talking to no one.

Then my friend Goedele invited me to a party. Gulya, as I called her, was a Belgian national who'd eventually marry my best friend, Bob. She was in Moscow teaching Russian to foreigners at the Anglo-American school. Gulya was filled with good-fellowship, energy, and charm. She enthused about everything, and was determined never to let the pressures of living in Moscow get her or her friends down.

The party was held at the home of one Martin Walker, a British journalist. No Russians were there. Just expats. With the exception of Goedele, I didn't know anyone. And nobody, not even Goedele, really knew me.

The music went on at ten o'clock. Rock-and-roll classics. Sixties and seventies gold. The Beatles. The

Stones. Crosby, Stills, Nash, and Young. When Gulya asked me if I'd like to dance, I returned in my mind to the wedding with Jeanette, to the dance floor with Lou Ginsberg's orchestra. And I remembered how good I'd felt that night, years before. And I surveyed the room and realized that nobody there at that British reporter's apartment knew that I didn't dance, that I couldn't dance, that I wouldn't dance, that I, Robert Rand, was a serious scholar of Soviet affairs, and therefore eschewed all movement to music. In short, there were, at that party, no expectations of how I should behave, and there would be, at that party, no stunned expressions should I throw off my jacket and dance.

As I pondered my options, Iris appeared, and her question of two years before taunted me, and dared me to act.

So I cut loose.

Gulya and I danced nonstop for three straight hours. Others danced that evening, too. But none with the passion that Gulya and I had. It was freestyle dancing. Jumping and hopping and twisting around like nobody ever in the Kremlin's shadow had jumped and hopped and twisted before. Arms pumping. Legs kicking. My body shook left and right and up and down as if it were coming apart. I grinned and sweated and grinned some more, and Moscow raised a bushy eyebrow, for it had never really seen me grin before. At one moment, sometime after midnight, I noticed that I was the only one dancing in that room, a lone, deranged, gleefully self-absorbed soul. By the time Goedele and I left the party, my clothing was drenched and my energy spent. And my mind was empty, its emotional gauge on calm, for I had experienced, for the first time ever, an epiphany of movement and music: the pure joy of dance.

Had I clung to the lesson I learned that evening, had I clutched it and nurtured it and made it part of my life, perhaps the disorder that had meddled with my mind would never have seized me again. But I returned home from Russia the same as before, as serious and intense as ever, and perhaps even more so, for I was jobless, and had much to prove.

3
Panic Attack

I spent my first year back from Moscow well removed from the dance floor, on fellowship at the Kennan Institute for Advanced Russian Studies in Washington, D.C.—a leading center of scholarship, a serious academic base whose mission was to ponder all things Russian. It was a wonderful place to think and to write. I received office space, money, and time to complete a book about law and crime and justice in Russia. The book told the story of a murder trial. That's what I'd followed while living in Moscow. Reviews of the work emphasized the serious nature of my scholarship. Nobody called it fun to read.

At the end of my Kennan fellowship, I landed a job as an editor at National Public Radio. NPR: the serious broadcasting network. Enormous prestige. Enormous pressure to succeed. Enormous satisfaction. Until one day—cruelly and quite without warning—the thing that had rattled my mental composure in Moscow returned with calamitous force.

It happened on December 7. Pearl Harbor Day. The attack came at work, during an editorial meeting. Chest pain. Rapid heartbeat. Nausea. An awful sense that needles were pricking at my head, that my mind had turned inside out.

I left the meeting prematurely, feeling unnerved and embarrassed. A colleague ran after me. My skin had turned ghost white, she said. She held my hand, which was pallid and cold.

At the emergency room an attendant said, "I see lots of sick people, and you look awfully sick." But the physicians could not find anything wrong. The EKG was normal. The chest pain was likely a simple muscle strain or bruised rib, they said. The early manifestations of my mental disorder were shadowy and ephemeral, masking their bite and intentions in unremarkable bodily functions. I was released on my own recognizance.

The ailment that had first appeared in Moscow refused to disappear. It was branded to the flesh of my subconsciousness and struck with increasingly terrible persistence. Day in and day out, for weeks at a time—episodes of sudden nausea, the racing heart, the imploded mind, a feeling that surely I would faint or, even worse, would die—all this poked and jabbed at my mind, like a matador stabbing a bull with barbed sticks, over and over again, the better to weaken his prey.

I struggled to get by, crawling through my days. The mornings were especially bad, for I feared what each day might bring. And since I was raised to be perfect, I took care to conceal my condition, for no one could know that a mental-health crisis had left me battered, then swallowed me whole. Me, the serious scholar turned serious editor. Me, the self-confident journalist whom colleagues much admired. The man who valued control had damn near totally lost it. I could not stomach the humiliation and stigma such a revelation would precipitate.

Nearly two years passed before I sought diagnosis and assistance. By then I had hit bottom. I barely got by. Work had become a nearly intolerable struggle in which, amidst the assaults of my physical symptoms, I battled to maintain some sense of poise and composure. I stopped seeing friends. I stopped dating women. I took pleasure in sleep and little more. Happiness, tranquility, joy—these became features of fiction. And dancing was the last thing on my mind.

From the *Diagnostic and Statistical Manual of Mental Disorders, Fourth Edition* (DSM-IV), American Psychiatric Association

PANIC ATTACK

A discrete period of intense fear or discomfort, in which four (or more) of the following symptoms develop abruptly and reach a peak within 10 minutes:
(1) palpitations, pounding heart, or accelerated heart rate
(2) sweating
(3) trembling or shaking
(4) sensations of shortness of breath or smothering
(5) feeling of choking
(6) chest pain or discomfort
(7) nausea or abdominal distress
(8) feeling dizzy, unsteady, lightheaded, or faint
(9) derealization (feelings of unreality) or depersonalization (being detached from oneself)

(10) fear of losing control or going crazy
(11) fear of dying
(12) paresthesias (numbness or tingling sensations)
(13) chills or hot flushes

From a pamphlet released by
the U.S. government's
National Institute of Mental Health

WHAT IS PANIC DISORDER?

In panic disorder, brief episodes of intense fear are accompanied by multiple physical symptoms (such as heart palpitations and dizziness) that occur repeatedly and unexpectedly in the absence of any external threat. These "panic attacks," which are the hallmark of panic disorder, are believed to occur when the brain's normal mechanisms for reacting to a threat—the so-called "fight or flight" response—becomes inappropriately aroused. Most people with panic disorder also feel anxious about the possibility of having another panic attack and avoid situations in which they believe these attacks are likely to occur. Anxiety about another attack, and the avoidance it causes, can lead to disability in panic disorder.

In the United States, between 3 and 6 million people will have panic disorder at some time in their lives. The disorder typically begins in young adulthood, but older people and children can be affected. Women are affected twice as frequently as men.

Typically, a first panic attack seems to come "out of the blue," occurring while a person is engaged in some ordinary activity like driving a car or walking to work. Suddenly, the person is struck by a barrage of frightening and uncomfortable symptoms. These symptoms often include terror, a sense of unreality, or a fear of losing control. This barrage of symptoms usually lasts several seconds, but may continue for several minutes. The symptoms gradually fade over the course of about an

31

hour. People who have experienced a panic attack can attest to the extreme discomfort they felt and to their fear that they had been stricken with some terrible, life-threatening disease or were "going crazy." Often people who are having a panic attack seek help at a hospital emergency room.

In panic disorder, panic attacks recur and the person develops an intense apprehension of having another attack. As noted earlier, this fear—called anticipatory anxiety or fear of fear—can be present most of the time and seriously interfere with the person's life even when a panic attack is not in progress. In addition, the person may develop irrational fears called phobias about situations where a panic attack has occurred. For example, someone who has had a panic attack while driving may be afraid to get behind the wheel again, even to drive to the grocery store.

People who develop these panic-induced phobias will tend to avoid situations that they fear will trigger a panic attack, and their lives may be increasingly limited as a result. Their work may suffer because they can't travel or get to work on time. Relationships may be strained or marred by conflict as panic attacks, or fear of them, rule the affected person and those close to them.

Panic disorder has been found to run in families, and this may mean that inheritance (genetics) plays a strong role in determining who will get it. Yet, many people who have no family history of the disorder develop it.

Although onset is known to be most frequent in adolescence and young adulthood, little is known about who is more likely to have an isolated attack, and, of those persons, who will go on to develop the full disorder, and what sequence of events may influence this. In this area, promising leads to follow are the investigation of temperament and personality; family and genetic patterns; developmental growth characteristics; and other biological, psychological, and environmental factors.

I first saw Dr. Steven Gilbert, a Washington, D.C., psychiatrist, in November 1991. He was referred by my internist, and I called him the day I reached inside myself and found nothing, absolutely nothing.

I had lost all semblance of self-confidence. My fear of panic attacks had become overwhelming. Anticipatory anxiety controlled every single aspect of my life, as surely as your lungs command your breath, or your eyes define your vision. Working, shopping, driving, socializing, even exercising—I gauged these activities by their potential to trigger uncontrollable, terrifying panic. There was much, very much, I didn't do for fear of bringing on attacks. I needed help.

By nature or design, Steve Gilbert really looked like a psychiatrist. He was slightly rumpled and a tad overweight, with the curly gray hair, glasses, and goatee you'd imagine a psychiatrist should have. He had the Harvard education, too. A couch was in his office, and his desk was topped with mounds of books and files and everyday riffraff that enhanced the impression that this was a fellow who cared about people and not about things.

His eyes struck me first, when I first went in to see him. They were friendly and compassionate eyes, to be sure, eyes that suggested a smile or laugh. But they were sad eyes, too, overlaid with a hint of melancholy, the toll from his patients' stories, I supposed, the toll from his years of practice.

At our first few sessions, Dr. Gilbert took stock of me. Here is what he wrote:

Ongoing saga of anxiety-stress-panic now major issue of life. Affects self confidence, ambitions. Socially things bad. Work——>Home——>Work. Wants to get monkey off back. Russia and USSR very important in life. Too serious. Intense.

Panic disorder, he said, was the clear diagnosis. We decided on a course of cognitive therapy. I would not take medication, for to do so, in my view, would have ceded control of my mind to some otherworldly substance. I valued control too much to do that. And I was still, even in my weakened state, the perfectionist I had always been: I would find a way within myself to understand and fix my problem. Dr. Gilbert would give me direction and guidance. But I would do it on my own.

The cure to my disorder, I discovered, in significant part was devilishly simple, at least in prescription. It was revealed after three months of therapy.

"You know," Dr. Gilbert said, "you are somebody who is very successful, and you've done a bunch of things that other people would kill to be able to do. Your career and your academic record have worked out very nicely, thank you very much. With nary a stumble. You're well respected. You have an interesting job. Good people to work with. Promotions. Responsibility. But you talk about these things without any sense of pleasure. You talk about having a book published at an incredibly young age, a book that was really well received and that was unique, and it sounds like it should have been this wonderful adventure pulling it together, except that you talk about it as if it were almost routine."

"Yeah, I guess," I said. "So what?"

"So when," Dr. Gilbert asked, "was the last time you had fun?"

I blinked at Dr. Gilbert, and turned my head away. It was a devastating question, really. A direct hit. I had no easy answer.

I sat there mute on his couch, stunned by the fact of my silence. And I reflected on his question—carefully, thoughtfully, soberly—for much was at stake; the answer brought me back three years, to that party in Moscow with Gulya, where I danced like an unleashed kangaroo. And before that, to the wedding with my old girlfriend Jeanette, where I sashayed my feet on the ballroom parquet, and jiggled my hips and snapped my fingers and even brandished a smile. And I realized that fun was so seldom a caller that I measured its visits by frequency in years.

"How sad," I thought. "How terribly, terribly sad."

Dr. Gilbert looked at me. I studied the floor, shaken, but aware—thanks to the jolt my psychiatrist had just delivered—that I had finally found a way to crawl out of my hole. Which brought me directly to Courtney Glass, my very first dance teacher, who saved my life.

4

Coco, the Dance Teacher

oco, as she preferred to be called, probably would have welcomed the opportunity to help mend my anxious mind, had I disclosed at the outset why I really wanted to meet her, why I needed to meet her. She was, I would discover, by nature a giver and a healer, one of those thoughtful people who looks after others better than themselves, a person for whom empathy and friendship mean everything. Family, she once told me, is a circle of friends who love you. As it was, she would learn of my struggle with panic disorder many months later, after we had cobbled together a friendship, after I had discovered that this slight, unsuspecting woman could literally steady in her arms—on the dance floor, of all places—my unsteady psyche, after she and I, by her own estimation, had become family.

Coco was born in Memphis and reared in Birmingham. The Alabama of her upbringing was, it seemed to me, a very anxious place—although she survived it just fine—a complicated slice of sixties and seventies American pie, a sweet-and-sour swirl of white versus black, of pride and of prejudice, of old and of new. Amidst the blend, three men stood out: George Wallace, the segregationist governor; Bear Bryant, the wildly popular

Crimson Tide football coach; and E.T., Coco's father. E.T., her favorite, was the one who knew how to dance.

E.T. jitterbugged, as most respectable dancers did back then, and as a child Coco would hop atop her daddy's shoes, grab his hands, and jitterbug as best she could. Father and daughter especially loved the lilting rhythms of a homespun tune about a local dance hall, "Tuxedo Junction." Popularized by Glenn Miller, the tune, composed in 1939 by Birmingham native Erskine Hawkins with lyrics by Buddy Feyne, was arguably the national anthem of the swing era. It was the soothing stuff, the state of mind, that Coco was raised on, and it predisposed her to the dance floor:

> Feelin' low, rockin' slow
> I want to go right back where I belong
> Way down South in Birmingham.
> I mean South in Alabam'
> There's an old place where people go
> To dance the night away.
> They all drive or walk for miles
> To get jive that southern style,
> It's an old jive that makes you want to dance
>   'till break of day.

For Courtney Glass, dancing was as familiar as the dawn cutting into day, and as pleasing and constant as the ebbing sun. It was, for her, a force of nature, a family bequest, something to treasure. For me, as Coco would eventually learn, dancing was aberrant, abnormal, eccentric, peculiar, and awfully frightening. I was drawn to dance, literally, out of panic and despair. Coco was drawn to dance because she had always done it, because she knew it to be good.

As a child Coco studied ballet. The movies later spurred her interest in social dance. "I was raised on Walt Disney films," she said, "on *Sleeping Beauty* and *Cinderella,* even *Gone with the Wind.* And there were in these films scenes of ballroom dancing, of women in long, beautiful dresses and handsome princes and swirling skirts and all the romance associated with that. And I was struck by it all, and to this day I carry the image of that in my head."

By the time she reached high school, Coco had learned how to "fish dance," as she called it, the wiggle-your-hips, arm-pumping, do-your-own-thing form of freestyle dancing associated with rock and roll. She also took to folk dancing, thanks to a summer's stay in Mexico with her mother, an anthropologist. That experience led her to join international folk dance groups during and after college. And that, in turn, turned her on to other forms of social dance: squares, contras, yet again swing, and, finally, Cajun.

It was through Cajun dancing that I first encountered Coco Glass. In the days after Dr. Gilbert posed his epiphanic question, I had resolved that I would take up social dancing, and Cajun, I decided, would be the dance form of choice. From the outset, it struck me as a bit absurd that I, a responsible journalist on the edge of middle age, an M.A., J.D., Russian-speaking Jewish guy with thinning brown hair from Chicago, would choose, of all things, Cajun dancing as an avocation. It was, quite literally, stuff from the other side of the planet. But the origins of the idea are simple enough and wholly withstand scrutiny: I had heard Beausoleil, the powerfully energetic Louisiana Cajun band, several times on the radio, and I liked their music very much. Their tunes moved me, and made me feel happy. And once, at a folk festival, I had seen Dewey Balfa, the icon of Cajun music and culture, and I liked him, too. So, I reasoned, if I was going to dance—and I knew I had to—Cajun seemed a legitimate course of treatment. And, like Bulgarian line dances, which I'd proved in my youth I could handle, Cajun dancing thrived on order, with steps and patterns I could study and master. It was, in short, a dance form of reason, a dance form for a serious man, like me, who was about to unleash a search for serious fun and sound mental health.

As for Coco, she had been in the Washington, D.C., area for more than ten years by the time I met her. She had her serious side, for she worked as a policy analyst and trainer for the federal government. But Coco became a fixture elsewhere, in the social dance community, where she was a leader on the dance floor. She organized swing dances and taught dance work- shops, helped out at summer dance camps, and at- tended just about every dance function there was. She also took up teaching Cajun dance after Twist and Shout, the blues club, began, in the mid-eighties, to book Louisiana bands. "I had the knack of breaking the steps down so they could be taught," she said.

Cajun music at the time was enjoying a renaissance that had attracted listeners well beyond Louisiana, including a core group of followers in Washington, D.C., among them Coco Glass. The music was well suited to Coco and her peers, the intelligentsia who labored by day in the nation's capital and played at night at Twist and Shout. The tunes were mostly bouncy, bright and cheerful, antidotes to the federal bureaucracy. As for the rhythms, they were infectious, virulently so, driven by the fiddle and the button accordion, a handheld squeeze box that appealed, in the grand tradition of nonpartisanship, to conservative and liberal sensibilities alike.

Coco learned how to Cajun dance from a French-speaking Cajun named Chris Trahan, a Twist and Shout regular who was born and raised in South Louisiana and who knew what he was doing. A bit of history, for Cajun music is steeped in it:

Chris's ancestors were the French Catholic pioneers who had settled in Nova Scotia in the early seventeenth century, in a region called Acadia. In 1713 France ceded this land to the British, who doubted the colonists' allegiance to the English Crown. In 1755 the British ordered the Acadians out of Nova Scotia. The expulsion, known in French as the *Grand Derangement*—the "Big Upheaval"—was, for these people, a paroxysm of history. It was also perhaps the first forced mass migration on the North American continent. The poet Henry Wadsworth Longfellow memorialized the event in *Evangeline,* his famous tale of lost lovers.

The Acadians, Longfellow wrote, were "scattered

like dust and leaves, . . . scattered were they, like flakes of snow." They wandered "friendless, homeless, hopeless . . . and many, despairing, heart-broken, asked of the earth but a grave."

Forced into exile, thousands of Acadians found their way to South Louisiana. There they became known as Cajuns. The southwestern part of the state—the Cajun hub, whose main population center is Lafayette—is still known locally as Acadiana.

Music and dance were and remain central to Cajun culture. Like Coco, and entirely unlike me, Chris Trahan learned how to dance as a child, "by observation," as he put it, at his mother's and grandmother's knees, at weddings or at other festive occasions when French-style music was performed, which was just about always and everywhere. As an adult Chris even worked for a time as a professional Cajun dancer, performing with dance troupes in the United States and abroad. He eventually moved to Baltimore to take a job in computers, his real trade. Twist and Shout, about forty-five minutes down the road, became his second home.

Coco first met Chris Trahan at a dance party of Twist and Shout regulars. "They put on some Cajun music," she said, "and there was this tall, dark-haired guy who was absolutely ripping up the dance floor. His arms were twirling and his feet were flying, and he was something to see. When the dance was over I said to him, 'I want you to teach me how to do that.'" He did, and Coco added Cajun to her dance-teaching portfolio.

I found Coco through the Washington Folklore Society, which sponsored local dances. "I'm looking for someone to teach me how to Cajun dance. Can you help me?" I asked. "Contact Coco Glass," they said.

When I telephoned Coco, she quickly agreed to take me on as a student. "You told me you loved Cajun music and had seen Dewey Balfa and had been so impressed that you wanted to learn how to dance to it. You sounded so nice, so I figured, let's give it a try."

I told her I was interested in private dance lessons, and not in her public workshops. I knew I'd be better able to handle the trauma of dancing, initially at least, in a closed setting, where Coco and Coco alone could see my mistakes. And should I, mid-lesson, succumb to a wave of anxiety, I would have to cower away from only one person.

Coco suggested we meet at her apartment one evening a week. Her fee was twenty dollars an hour.

On my way to see Coco the very first time, I had a panic attack. It came out of nowhere while I was driving my car at fifty-five miles an hour on the Capital Beltway, Washington's major highway. The assault was particularly vicious, taking hold of my head like a pincer, squeezing, once and then twice and then three times and four. Each contraction seemed intent on crumpling my mind.

I thought I would run off the road. I was traveling in the middle lane, trapped like a rat on a treadmill in what became, for the moment, a terrifying, unyielding flow of traffic. I squeezed hard on the steering wheel in search of stability, and of sanity. Tachycardia battered my heart. My head turned light. I sucked in a breath, and then spit it out. Inhale. Exhale. Inhale. Exhale. Fifteen seconds passed, although it seemed like minutes. The panic began to ease. It released its grip and went on its way. And although I was quite shaken, I continued to drive to my session with Coco. And in so doing, I broke through a wall, and my panic attacks didn't return quite so often anymore.

Dialogue with Dr. Steven Gilbert

ME: *The first time I told you about my interest in dancing was after I had just met Coco, and begun to dance. By that point in our therapy sessions, I had come, I think, to understand that I needed to find things in my life that would allow me to be a little boy, to be imperfect, to be silly. I think that's the word you used. Silly. The perfect antidote to perfection obsession. That's what you said silliness was.*

DR. GILBERT: *I remember that.*

ME: *And you had come up with a model, a clinical metaphor of sorts, that you used to help me understand my battle with panic disorder and, more to the point, to illustrate the way to treat it. Remember?*

DR. GILBERT: *It was the glass.*

ME: *It was the glass. You said, let's view the emotional self as a glass, and all life's emotions, good and bad, as water inside the vessel. And you said that as you go through life with all its stresses, your emotions will gradually rise to the top of the glass. And unless you do something to poke holes in the side, your emotional water will flood over the top and spill out, creating one big psychologically induced mess. And the result, in terms of everyday life, is malfunction, dysfunction, some form of disorder, some sort of chaos. Some people may have migraines. Some people may have irritable bowel syndrome. Some people may have ulcers. And I, thank you very much, had panic attacks.*

DR. GILBERT: *And you took the glass model and turned it into a challenge.*

ME: *Yes, and the challenge was to do something, to figure out how to poke holes into the side of the glass to allow all the stuff inside me to escape, to escape so I could breathe, so my emotions would be on an even keel. And one of the ways I did that was to learn how to have fun, to learn how to dance.*

DR. GILBERT: *But I recall that when you began to take dance lessons, you went about it seriously, ever the perfectionist. It began as an intellectual process for you, and not an emotional process.*

Because all your life, what you had was a series of intellectual successes, but not joy. What was lacking in you was an inner voice that said, "Hey, way cool!"

ME: *Yeah, you're right. I was pretty intense about learning how to dance, and learning how to dance just right. I went at it dead-stone serious.*

DR. GILBERT: *But like most athletic challenges, in order to get good you have to be willing to make mistakes. There's no way to step from the clamshell, fully clothed, fully competent, onto the dance floor. You just can't do it. And so to get good at it you have to be willing to be inept, to be clumsy, to not know what you're doing, literally to step on other people's toes. And if you're lucky you have teachers who accept that and are willing to tolerate that. Someone who's willing to say, "Of course he's not good at this. But that's okay."*

ME: *Well, I found that one person, and it was Coco.*

There are many firsts in life, and most are not moments of derring-do or of high drama. Instead, like a trigger, they set something in motion, the payoff, in due course, to follow. A first date may lead to a first kiss, which may develop into love, which may produce a marriage, which may produce a family. At the end of the day, something truly grand has been accomplished. But at the beginning, at the first step, a great sense of moment or of import does not, by itself, attach. And so it was for me, as I stood at Coco's doorstep, about to join her school of Cajun dance.

I was anxious, to be sure, as any new student in any new classroom with any new teacher might be. But, curiously, not overly anxious, despite my panic attacks, despite my lifelong fear of dance. Instead, by the time I had reached Coco's apartment, I had settled myself and was focused and resolved. My first dance lesson was to be a challenge, like many I had faced throughout my career, and I would be its master. I was, to continue the schoolhouse analogy, determined to ace the exam. In fact, I entered Coco's apartment very much the diligent student, with a pen and pad of paper tucked inside the pocket of my shirt, the better to take notes on whatever Coco had to say. The notion of fun had not yet affected the enterprise at hand.

"You weren't real relaxed," Coco later recalled. "My first impression was this is a pretty shy guy. You looked a little bashful. You didn't talk a lot. But you were wearing a flannel shirt, and I appreciated guys in flannel, so I figured you'd be okay."

Coco, I learned, was a wonderful teacher. She was, above all, welcoming, with green eyes and chipmunk-like cheeks and a mischievous grin that set me at ease while setting me straight. At first introduction, you couldn't really pick up on her Alabama roots. Her drawl had thinned a bit after years of working up north, in or around the federal government. But the gentility was still there: the warmth of a Birmingham August still stoked her smile, and her eyes, those bright green eyes, had a kind and easy-going way about them, a southern sparkle I found pleasing, like mint to iced tea.

Coco was patient, as if she had never met a man with two left feet she didn't like. And she had a way, with language, of making the most difficult dance steps understandable. She likened the Cajun jig, a one-step dance with an up-and-down motion, to "walking along the street with one foot on the curb and the other in the gutter." And the Cajun two-step became a simple matter of moving my legs, left foot then right, in a "step-together, step-touch" pattern.

Week after week, Coco would walk me through these patterns, slowly and patiently, until they made sense. Her technique as a teacher was easy to follow: she instructed by induction, where particular steps produced a whole. A dance, she said, consisted of component parts. Layer one basic element on top of another— one step, then one weight shift, then one arm lead, then one turn—and eventually the dance would appear. It was pure chemistry, as sure, she maintained, to draw out the dancer in me as two parts of hydrogen and one of oxygen were certain to produce water. Her approach appealed to the analytical nature of my mind. If I mastered the basics, I could perfect the dance.

We tackled the two-step first. "It's the dance the Cajuns are most proud of," Coco said.

It began with my standing in place, knees flexed, on her living room parquet floor, bobbing slowly up and down, like a buoy on water, in search of rhythm.

"Listen to the music," Coco said. A slow accordion tune presented the challenge. Something called "Coeur des Cajuns" (Heart of the Cajuns):

> *La joie de vivre c'est dans l'accordéon,*
> *La joie de vivre c'est dans les belles chansons,*
> *La musique c'est une tradition*
> *Et c'est dans les coeurs de tous les Cajuns.*

> [The joy of life is in the accordion,
> The joy of life is in the beautiful songs,
> The music is a tradition
> And it's in the hearts of all the Cajuns.]

The tune was written by Bruce Daigrepont, an accordionist from New Orleans. "Bruce is my favorite," Coco said. She closed her eyes and listened to the music, pinching the middle finger of her right hand against her right thumb, as if she were going to snap out the beat. The snap never came, as if snapping would show disrespect. She instead bounced her right arm, along with her body, silently UP and DOWN, in pace with the lyrics of the song: "La JOIE / de VIVRE / c'est DANS / l'accordéON, / La JOIE / de VIVRE / c'est DANS / les belles chansONS."

"You've got to find the beat before you can dance," Coco said. "Feel the rhythm. ONE, two, THREE, four. STEP-together, STEP-touch."

"Say it," she demanded.

"ONE, two, THREE, four. STEP-together, STEP-touch," I replied. All the while I lurched at the knees,

49

UP at one and then DOWN at two and then UP at three and then DOWN at four.

"The knee bends are part of the posture of the Cajun two-step," she said. "It's a subtle point, but important to get in there early."

After the knee bobs, Coco suggested I actually walk through the dance. I was to move—in STEP-together, STEP-touch choreography—to a ONE-TWO-THREE-four beat.

"Watch my feet, and you follow," Coco said, positioning in front of me, her back to my face. "First we'll just go to the left. Follow me: STEP-together, STEP-touch. STEP-together, STEP-touch. LEFT-together, LEFT-touch. LEFT-right, LEFT-right.

"Okay. Now let's move in the other direction: RIGHT-together, RIGHT-touch. RIGHT-together, RIGHT-touch. RIGHT-left, RIGHT-left. RIGHT-together, RIGHT-touch."

Obligingly, with each step and together and left and right, I shuffled my feet on the floor. I struggled, at Coco's urging, to maintain a concurrent up-and-down movement. But my brain, which had never before simultaneously moved laterally and vertically, rebelled.

"It's hard," I said, flustered, glaring at my feet.

I spent most of that first lesson, and much time during many subsequent sessions, glaring at my feet.

"Don't worry, you'll get it," Coco said. "Your body just needs to get used to it. After a while, muscle memory will kick in."

I was struck by the phrase.

"It's when dancing becomes a reflex," Coco said. "Your legs will move naturally, and you won't even think about it. And when you stop thinking and start dancing with muscle memory, that's when the fun begins."

The actual two-step dance, Coco said, called for stringing together left and then right pairs of STEP-together, STEP-touches, as in LEFT-together, LEFT-touch / RIGHT-together, RIGHT-touch. Each STEP-together, STEP-touch (the fundamental "two-step" unit) was to be executed at forty-five-degree angles: first, two steps to the left at forty-five degrees, then two steps to the right at forty-five degrees. In that manner, Coco explained, the two steps would propel me forward zigzag style through the line of dance. "Remember, forty-five degrees," she said. "And always counterclockwise. The line of dance is always counterclockwise around the dance floor."

Straightforward rules. No room for improvisation. The two-step had appeal.

Next in the lesson came the placement of feet vis-à-vis your partner. "Staggered," Coco said, turning toward me. "Not lined up together. Our toes should be staggered. That way our legs won't bang into each other."

Thus aligned, she engaged me, without warning, in the ballroom position. "Your left hand takes my right hand and holds it out so," she said, thrusting our opposing arms outward toward the wall. My grip was uncertain. "No spaghetti arms," she said. "Hold me firm enough to give tension, but not so strong as to

overpower. And place your other hand around here"—
she took my right palm and plastered it to a spot
underneath her left shoulder blade. Suddenly, Coco
and I were fully attached. It was, for me, an awkward
moment. I was not accustomed to holding strange
women in my arms. For Coco, however, it was mechanical, a utilitarian joining of bodies, wholly devoid
of emotional content, for the sole purpose of con-
structing a four-legged vehicle to move around the
dance floor. That was the way of partner dancing, and
I'd have to get used to it.

With "Coeur des Cajuns" still on the stereo, we
began to move, counterclockwise, zigzagging left and
then right, across the wooden tiles of Coco's living room
floor. Her grip on me was steady, and her direction clear.
And so it would go, week after week, until she was certain that I had gotten it, and that I was, in fact, dancing.
And with each session I gained confidence, the very
thing that panic disorder had stripped me of. With
Coco, anxiety seemed to wane, at least in her apartment. It was a sanctuary as much as a dance floor.

Once I had the two-step down, Coco went on to
the jig. "I also call it the one-step, or jitterbug. It's a
more energetic dance, done to faster music."

On went a CD. A song called "Bosco Stomp." "I
just love this one," Coco said. It would become a favorite of mine, too. The tune was bright and quick and ut-
terly uplifting.

The one-step is a relatively new form of Cajun dance, its origins found in silliness and spontaneity, exactly the things I needed. According to Barry Jean Ancelet, a professor of folklore and Francophone studies at the University of Louisiana at Lafayette, it was created out of happenstance, born from some tongue-in-cheek chicanery at a Lafayette club in the mid-1970s.

"I was there," Ancelet said. "There was a man named Leroy Evans, and he was a great dancer. Quite popular with the women. And he showed up at this dance one day with a twisted ankle. He didn't want to dance, but the women made him do it anyway. He dragged his foot around, limping to the music. We thought it was hilarious and imitated him. Soon enough, everybody started doing it. Next thing you know it was the dance of a generation."

The one-step, Ancelet quipped, was originally called "Poor Leroy Can't Dance."

Coco explained that the one-step was later embellished at Mulate's, a dance hall in Breaux Bridge, by some of Chris Trahan's friends. They added intricate leads and arm formations, ruffles and flourishes that came from a hodgepodge of sources, including standard American jitterbug swing, Fred Astaire movies, and international folk dance.

The one-step required a more pronounced up-and-down motion than the two-step. "It does resemble limping," Coco said. "Remember the analogy about walking with one-foot-on-the curb and one-foot-in-the-gutter. Keep your weight on your left leg and place it on the curb. Bend it a bit. Then step with your right leg down into the gutter. Then back to the left again." The goal was to produce a pistonlike up-down, straight-drop pumping motion.

My introduction to the one-step began with marching orders. "Straight, drop, straight, drop, straight, drop, straight, drop," Coco said, while showing me the step. "You can do it, sweetie."

She grabbed my hands, turned toward me, and urged me to follow along. "Just try to feel the rhythm and move up and down with me."

Straight, drop, straight, drop. Up, down, up, down. Drop, straight, straight, drop. Down, up, down, down. The leg work was torturous. Again, my brain rebelled. But "Bosco Stomp" had hit a button, and I wanted to nail this dance.

We worked on the jig for many, many weeks. After each lesson, I'd go home and turn on the stereo and practice, hours at a time, one-stepping up and down in front of a full-length mirror until my thighs ached. I jigged at first to "Bosco Stomp," which I had dubbed from Coco's CD. Then I jigged to a song from Michael Doucet, Beausoleil's lead singer. His fiddle was solid and his lyrics true: *O yaie, bébé, O yaie, catin, O yaie, 'tit monde tu m'as fait du mal.* "O yaie, babe, O yaie, girl, O yaie, little world you've done me wrong."

One evening, when I was at Coco's, she decided to drill me in a really fast-paced jig. By then, I'd pretty much mastered the leg-pumping motion of the dance, and I'd even learned a few special leads. So once the music was on and we started to move, I was able to use my arms to spin her around me, and to spin us both around the center point of dance like a tight little fixed tornado. And there was a moment that evening when, finally, it clicked, and I realized my partner and I were dancing together as one, almost effortlessly, in time with the music.

I clung to that moment and lingered there, for it felt good; and as I held on, I took Coco and spun her again, spontaneously and with uncharacteristic precision, speed, and grace, around and around and around. And quite without thinking, in the midst of this twirling, I smiled, then giggled. And Coco giggled, too. And my giggle turned into laughter, loud and fresh and unimpeded. The last time I had felt that good was in Moscow, four years before, when Gulya and I rock-and-rolled. It was the lightest, best, most carefree moment I had experienced since panic disorder had knocked me off balance and sullied my outlook on life. I felt gleeful, like a toddler who'd been tickled silly in the ribs. It was cathartic. It was fun. And it was a giant stride ahead on the road to my recovery.

5

ISO Dance-Floor
Perfection

*

Dialogue with Dr. Steven Gilbert

DR. GILBERT: *What is important about dancing is that when you're focusing on getting the muscle memory, it's hard to worry about the other stuff. When you're on the dance floor, all you're thinking about is getting it right. Figuring out where the left foot should go next. And where the right foot should go after that.*

ME: *So you're not thinking about having a panic attack.*

DR. GILBERT: *You're not thinking about having a panic attack. Your thinking is centered. It's "Gee, how do I do this? What do I do next? Where's the rhythm? Where's the beat?"*

ME: *And gradually you get it right, and you begin to enjoy the music, and you begin to enjoy the whole experience of moving on a dance floor. And then your world off the dance floor seems a whole lot better, too. And then all of a sudden you're operating at a whole different level of life.*

DR. GILBERT: *And that's where the wheels leave the ground.*

57

The idea took shape within days of the "night of the Cajun giggle," as Coco described our Cajun-jig epiphany. It was, in hindsight, an absurd scheme. Only an earnest, wide-eyed, half-cocked proselyte dancer could have concocted it. But there it was, nonetheless. The perfect plan. The ultimate antianxiety prescription.

The dancing bug had nipped me good. Having conquered the Cajun jig, I might as well have scaled Everest. There was nothing, I decided, no twist, no turn, no spin, no pirouette, that I couldn't master. I would, I resolved, become the dancer's dancer. King of the ballroom. No matter I had never actually gone to a dance, or danced with anyone other than Coco. I was on a rampage—gotta dance, gotta dance!—and be it resolved that no tango nor salsa nor Irish jig would sidestep the tracks of my newfound dancing feet. I would, simply put, learn how to dance everything. And once I had done it, I would take Coco out on the town and teach her how to move.

Step one.

I began with Scottish country dancing.

I wasn't quite sure what Scottish country dancing was, but I knew that a course was offered at a community center near Coco's house, and, more to the point, I really liked Scottish music. If I'd learned one thing from my lessons with Coco, it's that you've got to love the music you dance to. The fiddle and bagpipe, mainstays of the Scottish band, moved me nearly as much as the fiddle-accordion blend in a Cajun ensemble.

I telephoned the instructor in advance of my arrival.

"Hi," I said, "I'm interested in Scottish country dancing. Do you take beginners?"

"Yes, of course," a female voice replied. "We welcome everyone to our community. We meet on Tuesday nights."

"It's partner dancing, right?"

"Yes."

"And you dance to the fiddle and bagpipe?"

"Yes. Why don't you come? I'm sure you'll enjoy it."

The next Tuesday evening, I drove up to the building where Scottish country dancing took place. It was dark outside. As I approached, I saw two men in kilts, lingering by the entrance. A third man in a kilt, even more foreboding, was lurking up a nearby road.

Oh, laddie. Dancing was challenging enough without the tartan accoutrements. If kilts were part of Scottish country dancing, then Scottish country dancing would not be part of me.

I went home.

Step two.

Merengue.

I had dated a Latina woman once, who hailed from Central America. She liked to dance, but had never imposed her habit on me, at least not while we were together. We parted as friends, so I called her up.

"Teach me that dance you do," I said.

The next evening, she was in my living room, jogging her elbows and jutting her hips left and then right as she stepped about a circle. I had, to be sure, seen her buttocks before, but never before had I seen her buttocks, or anyone else's, move quite in that way. It was brazen and melodic and oh so very, very feminine.

"Cuban motion," she said. "Try it."

I demurred. "No way," I said.

End of lesson.

Step three.

The Lindy Hop.

I knew Thea and John through my Russian connections. John spoke Russian better than any American I had ever met. His wire-rimmed glasses and bushy beard lent a Tolstoyan sort of credibility to his flawless Cyrillic accent. Thea spoke Russian, too, but she, a lean, pleasing woman with long brown hair, preferred to dance. And she did so, with John, at least once a week. Her favorite was the Lindy Hop, an eight-count explosion of jazz and swing that *Life* magazine once called America's folk dance. The Lindy was named after Charles Lindbergh, and the Hop described its capacity to fly. Thea had her aviator's wings, so I asked her and John to give me a lesson.

After dinner one evening at their Capitol Hill apartment, my friends rolled up the living room rug.

"You know, Rob," Thea said, "this is a pretty difficult dance. I don't think it's for a beginner."

"Just show me what it's like," I insisted.

What followed was the most amazing demonstration of dance-floor artistry I had ever witnessed. With some big-band music on the stereo, Thea and John joined in the closed position and simply took off. Their skill left me stunned. They circled each other once and then twice at incorrigible speed, and then bolted apart, still joined at the arm. In that open position they frolicked and kicked, and then closed in again, like a rubber band snapping, for some more of the circles. A flurry of moves ensued with names from another era: Charlestons, Suzy-Qs, slip slops, peck pecks.

When they'd finished, they were sweating, and I was puffed up with enthusiasm.

"I gotta learn how to do that!" I said. In my mind's eye I saw myself dancing with Coco, in command, strong of lead, firm of grip, impressing the hell out of all who would see us. Master of the ballroom. The perfect social dancer. Goddammit. That's what I'd become. The Cajun jig. The Lindy Hop. I'd do it all.

Thea smiled and looked at John. Then she looked at me.

"You should first learn how to swing."

Step four.

My local ballroom dance studio. This, I figured, was the very best way to go. Professional assistance from professional instructors. A serious course of study. Here I could tackle a range of social dance forms, from the fox-trot to the rumba, and I could do it privately, with a minimum of embarrassment, on my own time, at my own pace. The perfect means to implement my plan. I couldn't wait to get going. Lindy Hop, here I come.

One phone call and a free introductory lesson was mine for the taking. My guide for the afternoon: a certain Miss Cindy, former Class AA All–East Coast Open Mambo and PasoDoble champion, or something like that. Her mission for the hour: to teach me how to six-count swing.

"We'll begin with the swing because it's the most versatile of social dances," she said. "You can do it to rock and roll. You can do it to disco. You can do it at parties. You can do it at weddings. If you know how to swing, every girl will want to dance with you."

"Sounds good," I said.

Cindy was tall, slim, blond, and sequined. She wore high heels and red lipstick. Her hair was coiffed and sprayed, and a cloud of perfume enveloped her torso. Her eyes had an inorganic quality, as if sucked dry from boredom, or from one too many novice dancers. Her demeanor was polite but distant. Her voice was sharp, and a bit intimidating.

"Ever dance?" she asked.

"Of course," I said, nodding my head. "Cajun."

I was feeling cocky. "Two-step. Jig. And," I added enthusiastically, "a little bit of waltz." That was my latest endeavor with Coco.

"We don't do country-western here," she said. "Ever swing dance?"

"No. But I'd like to learn how to Lindy Hop."

"Let's begin."

She walked to a portable CD player and turned on some music. It was something unfamiliar, synthesized rock and roll with an edge of disco. Ballroom Mantovani. I grimaced.

"Robert," Cindy said, "we're going to do two triple steps and a rock step."

She paused, waiting for some grunt of acknowledgment, some trace of recognition. There was none forthcoming. There were no triple steps nor rock steps in the two-step, jig, or Cajun waltz.

"Two triple steps and a rock step," she repeated. "It goes like this: LEFT-right-left, RIGHT-left-right, rock back. ONE-two-three, FOUR-five-six, rock back. TRIP-le-step, TRIP-le-step, rock back. It's the foundation of the six-count swing."

I stared at her spiked feet as they rushed through the pattern. I had no idea what she was doing.

"Now you try it."

I stood there, disabled, feeling nervous and quite vulnerable. I didn't want to look like a fool, but I saw no way around it. Then, as those who have lived with panic disorder often tend to do, at moments of uncertainty, I switched my mind to rerun and revisited the past. Flashes went off in my brain. Memories of panic attacks. Recollections of similar times when control and perfection gave way to reality. A finger of anxiety jabbed at my stomach. It startled me, like a pop in the solar plexus. I wobbled in silence, trying to gauge what was going on. After a few seconds, I regained my focus.

"Could you please repeat that?" I asked.

"LEFT-right-left, RIGHT-left-right, rock back. TRIP-le-step, TRIP-le-step, rock back. You try it, please."

When done properly, the triple step can make a dancer pulse with rhythm. The rock step, in which the body juts back on the left foot then forward on the right, can hammer home a dance formation, like an exclamation point. When done improperly, the triple step–rock step combination can make you look like I looked, standing there in front of Cindy, stomping stiffly left and right, as if I were teetering on stilts. I was wooden-legged and well off beat. There was no pulse to my motion. There was no exclamation point. There was just pathetic. Plus humiliation.

She grabbed at my arms as a mother would pull at a fidgety child. "Just follow me," she said. I was cut by her edge of impatience. "LEFT-right-left, RIGHT-left-right, rock back. ONE-two-three, FOUR-five-six, rock back. TRIP-le-step, TRIP-le-step, rock back. Come on."

And so it went. I gamely—obediently—tried to mirror her image. But all I could manage were stumbles and slips. And with each misstep, the anxiety within me welled.

"TRIP-le-step, TRIP-le-step, rock back. TRIP-le-step, TRIP-le-step, rock back."

I was feeling woozy and lightheaded. What if I

actually had a panic attack? Would I be able to cover it up? What if I fainted? Or threw up? How could I get out of here? All the old feelings returned on the heels of Cindy's triple step.

Finally, the lesson ended. Cindy directed me to her office.

"I really need to go," I said.

She handed me a brochure. "We offer six weeks of lessons with one Saturday-night social party for one hundred twenty dollars. Or you can save some money by signing up for a ten-week course with two evening socials for one seventy-five. Which one would you prefer?"

"Well, I'd really like to think about it."

"These prices won't last long, you know."

"Thanks. But I'll get back to you."

"Robert, I think you would really benefit from the six-week course. And the social provides a great opportunity to meet the ladies."

With brochure in hand, I got up and fled the building.

Step five: Dr. Gilbert.

Dialogue with Dr. Steven Gilbert

ME: *I don't understand why it happened. I mean,
I'd been feeling well for weeks and weeks. Coco*

and I were doing great. No panic attacks. Very little anxiety. I was even having fun. I thought I had beaten the thing. And then all of a sudden at this stupid dance lesson I started to feel out of control. It was very discouraging.

DR. GILBERT: I'm not surprised.

ME: What do you mean?

DR. GILBERT: Well, I probably should have told you to expect it. I call it picking the scab.

ME: What do you mean, "picking the scab"?

DR. GILBERT: Look, you had been fighting with your problem for years. You'd been bruised and scratched. Finally, you turned the corner and started to heal. Those scratches turned into scabs. And what do people do when they have scabs?

ME: They pick at them.

DR. GILBERT: Uh-huh.

ME: So you mean it was natural that I'd somehow revisit my panic problem, that I'd somehow pick at it, in your words?

DR. GILBERT: Absolutely.

ME: Lenin had another way of saying it, you know. One step backward, two steps forward. The revolution would steadily progress, he said, but not without setbacks. So I guess you're saying that I should have expected my recovery to go the same way?

DR. GILBERT: *That's right. In the realm of psychiatric therapy, things progress slowly. What takes the rest of the world one week to accomplish will take us a year. We call it shrink time.*

6

Life on the Dance Floor

S o. My blitzkrieg on the ballroom didn't work. The scheme proved to have been ill-conceived and harebrained, like earth shoes or eight-tracks or the Mike Dukakis presidential campaign. Great ideas all, fueled as they were by zeal and by good intentions. But they lacked in smarts and in foundation, and so did my rush to the dance floor. I simply didn't have the legs, or the experience, to swing or to Lindy Hop. Nor, I discovered, had I overcome bouts with anxiety and panic.

I had stupidly told Coco about my plans to master every dance there is, to appear one day on her doorstep to sweep her off her feet in a flurry of tango and fox-trot and jitterbug finesse. She had responded with understated amusement to the notion, raising an eyebrow just a tad, no doubt ascribing my enthusiasm to the hysteria a beginner can bring to any new passion in life. But Coco loved to dance so much that she never belittled my enterprise. She once even offered to teach me a swing step or two. We never got that far, however. Triple-Step Cindy had intervened.

So back to the basics. I focused again on my lessons with Coco, and withdrew to the familiar ground of Cajun dance.

By that time Coco and I had become friends. She stopped accepting payment for our weekly get-togethers. "I enjoy this too much to take your money," she said. Our sessions stretched to three hours: one hour of dance, then two hours of talk. She'd feed me cookies and chamomile tea. I'd bring along the occasional bottle of wine. I wondered whether she might have developed a crush on me, or I a crush on her.

One evening, not long after the Triple-Step–Cindy affair, I told Coco about my panic disorder.

"It made me feel sad for you," she said. "And it made me feel closer to you, too. I always have a kinship for people who are working on things, so I could relate to your need to talk stuff out. I was surprised that someone like you who was so intelligent and successful, someone with so many impressive credentials, would find himself with those kinds of troubles. I was surprised because it seemed to me that all of the positive things you had going for you should have supported your self-confidence, and it's the lack of self-confidence that should be the basis of emotional problems. You had plenty to be self-assured about, whereas I, a mere mortal, should have been more susceptible to such things."

Coco's reaction surprised me, for she had it upside down. Self-confidence may have led to whatever successes I had in life, but the pursuit of success, for me at least, had a chronic, unhealthy constitution. There was, in Dr. Gilbert's words, no "way cool" feeling to lubricate the ride. Anxiety and panic had intervened, and self-confidence, that font of creativity and professional achievement, had all but vanished. But Coco, for all her so-called mere mortality, knew how to have fun. "I work to live, I don't live to work," she once told me. I didn't completely buy her philosophy of life, but I knew her well enough and admired her sense of play and of joy to appreciate the point. And the point, in terms of the challenge at hand, was for me to get out of her living room studio and onto a genuine dance floor, with bona fide dancers and all that might entail.

So at Coco's urging, I resolved to go to Cherry Hill, a trailer-park dance hall in College Park, Maryland. The place was an aberration in Washington terms. Tucked just inside the Beltway a half hour's drive from Capitol Hill, Cherry Hill's lots were bustling with mobile homes and itinerant Winnebagos. There wasn't a Brooks Brothers' suit to be found. This was where the real America bedded down for the night, the cross-country travelers from Maine or Nebraska come, for a day or two, to see their nation's capital. At the edge of the park was a recreation hall, with washers and dryers, a food stand, and dance floor. Cleanliness, sustenance, and social dance: this was the Cherry Hill vision of what the country really cared about.

Cajun bands played at Cherry Hill every Friday night, and each week, before the band struck up, Coco would offer an hour-long beginning Cajun workshop. My plan was to take her workshop, then ease into the dance.

I had trouble working on the day of my first trip to Cherry Hill. Fridays at National Public Radio were pretty intense, for the show that I edited aired on the weekend, and Fridays offered a last chance to prepare, in relative calm, for what might lie ahead. There was always much to do. Interviews to tape. Pieces to cut down to size. Copy to hammer out. Weekend news coverage to arrange. It was late winter of 1992, and the presidential primaries had begun. George Bush Sr. was worrying about Pat Buchanan. Bill Clinton's worry was Gennifer Flowers. The country was worried about Iraq, which had just lost a war but was still acting up. And the IRA was bombing London. We were supposed to cover it all. But all I could think of was Beausoleil, and all day long an accordion tune bounced around my head. Journalism notwithstanding, my maiden Cajun dance was coming up, and it was, indisputably, the lead story.

I was, at one level, truly excited about my first dance. I had prepared for the day for weeks, and knew it was time to test out on the dance floor what I had practiced at Coco's apartment. And I really looked forward to asking Coco to two-step, waltz, and jitterbug with a genuine Cajun band providing the music. But I also felt considerable apprehension. This was, in a sense, another first day of school, and I was the panic-stricken eight year old the teacher would haul to the front of the class and introduce as new. All the kids' eyes would focus on me. What would they be thinking? What would they be like? Would I be made to feel welcome? Would anyone other than Coco want to dance with me? Would I, in fact, be able to dance? Would all of those hours at Coco's apartment translate into dance-floor poise and lead me to have fun? Or would I be kicked to the curb, a victim of the real world of social Cajun dance?

As I headed to Cherry Hill, anxiety reared up. I chewed and destroyed the inside of my cheek.

My first dance, like the others that soon followed, proved to be a difficult affair. The workshops themselves weren't too bad. All I had to do was silently stand there and follow Coco's orders. And since these were beginning sessions, I already knew the basic steps.

At a typical workshop Coco would ask all her students to partner up.

"Y'all don't be shy," she'd holler. "Find yourselves a buddy. If you don't have one, raise your hands."

Once we were all paired off, Coco would teach us a move, layering, as was her style, one component on top of another. After we'd practiced with our partners, Coco would ask us to rotate and try out the move with another student. No two people dance alike, she said, so changing partners would broaden our horizons and make us better dancers.

I loved the order and efficiency of these teaching sessions, and was, in these endeavors, a strong and active leader. I had, after all, been through these steps before. Little chance here of my screwing up or presenting myself as a fool. So as we changed partners I found myself asserting an air of command, directing women less confident than I through the familiar step-together, step-touch of the two-step, or the up-down, foot-in-the-gutter gyrations of the Cajun jig. These moments made me feel secure, and maybe even arrogant, for I, unlike the other greenhorns, knew what I was doing.

"No, no," I once said to an attractive if unsteady young lady who was struggling through the two-step. "Listen to what Coco says. You've got to bend your knees when you move across the floor."

When the band took the stage, however, and the real dance commenced, my confidence tucked tail and scampered away. The workshop had been my safety net, a nonthreatening platform on which I had some power and control. The actual event was a different affair, an arena of chaos and free-market forces in which only the fittest survived. Once the dancing began, that same young lady I had tried to instruct was never alone for a two-step or waltz. Good-looking women, I'd soon discover, rarely lacked for eager partners. I, on the other hand, played the role of the reticent wallflower, a fragile and timid and wilting little daffodil too scared to ask strangers to dance but too proud to let on that I cared.

Notwithstanding all that I had been through, and notwithstanding all that I had learned, both from Coco and from Dr. Gilbert, the actual act of stepping out was awfully hard to realize. So I stood there for most of my earliest dances, like a folding chair, arms intertwined across my chest, back rigid, face unsmiling, propped against the wall.

It was all quite intimidating.

At each of these venues, thirty or forty dancers would show up. "Regulars," is what Coco called them. They were big-time hoofers in the major leagues: a skilled, experienced, unforgiving group. After the band of the evening had turned on its mikes and the first reedy notes of a Cajun accordion jumped from the stage, these dancers would pair up and two-step or waltz, en masse, in a dizzying current of motion that flowed counterclockwise around the dance floor. On the fast tunes, jitterbuggers would fill the ballroom's center, pivoting madly, like two-person tops. The dancers all moved with speed and conviction and grace. And they took no prisoners: if you knew what to do, you were welcomed; if you didn't, you were ignored.

I was ignored, despite Coco's efforts. "Hey, y'all," she said to a group of her friends midway through my Cherry Hill debut. "This is Rob, and he's a student of mine and he's taking lessons from me, and I hope you-all will dance with him and welcome him to our community."

Her appeal went unheeded. Which was just as well, considering my trepidation. I was, in effect, a foreign tourist at Cherry Hill, visiting a place whose language I really barely spoke, and whose culture I didn't know at all. Coco was there, to be sure—my interpreter, so to speak—and I felt confident enough to invite her to dance, for I knew she'd say yes, and I knew she'd treat me gently, for she had seen all my errors before. And while dancing with her that evening, when I'd falter by missing a step or by losing a lead, she would gracefully take the dance over, preserving and steadying the base of our partnership, and saving us both from a stumbling indignity.

Which is one way to say there were no magic moments in my very first outing with Coco at Cherry Hill. I held her, yes, and we moved to music. And in that sense we danced. But my muscles had not memorized any semblance of routine. Out on the dance floor with her, I simply didn't know what to do next. Yes, I could step-together, step-touch, and even execute the up-and-down flow of the Cajun jig. But what could I do to make it more interesting? Social dancing—good social dancing—involves seamless patterns of moves and direction, a game plan of sorts, that propel the couple through their encounter with diversity and style and verve and panache. All I could offer Coco were miscues of various stripes and degrees. And lots and lots of hesitation, as I'd stop, literally, in my tracks, to ponder what the hell I was doing. It was, for me, a genuine struggle. And for Coco, I imagined, it must have been like being stuck in the grasp of a painfully tedious movie.

"I remember two-stepping around the dance floor with you that first time at Cherry Hill," Coco later recalled. "And I remember your trying really hard and being really self-conscious and stiff. You really were. But I also remember your tenacity. You were determined to get it, and you worked real hard at it. I could see that on your face. But I think at that point you were having to work too hard. You weren't having fun."

No kidding. And things got worse at my very first dances when I entertained the notion of engaging a partner other than Coco.

It was difficult, *really* difficult, to muster the courage to ask anyone else to dance. It's not that I couldn't approach strange women. It's just that I couldn't approach strange women dancers whose skill surpassed mine. I didn't have the vocabulary. They were behemoths. I was a rookie. They wanted dance-floor fireworks and footwork perfection, at least so I thought. I offered doubt, apprehension, fumbling, and fear.

Coco was sensitive to my concerns. And at every dance she'd continue the courtesy of introducing me to her friends, many of them women, and gradually they would agree, some reluctantly, some not so, to jitterbug or waltz, even though I was a beginner. Sometimes the experience was nice, and the women quite patient as I walked them around the circle of dance, exhausting my small lexicon of moves. Sometimes, if I screwed up, the dancing was ugly, and the women rude. Once, during a waltz, I lost track of the beat. My partner, a good-looking lady with years of Cajun dance in her feet, tossed me a venomous look and hammered me hard on the right shoulder, trying, with force, to push me back on track. I was stunned and embarrassed.

Another time a seasoned dancer, having consented

to put up with me, stopped the dance midstream. "This just isn't working out," she said.

And then there were the rejections.

"Would you like to dance?" I asked.

"No, thanks."

"How about you? Would you like to dance?"

"No, I don't think so. I've never seen you around here."

"Excuse me, would you care to two-step?"

"Well, you're a beginner, right?"

"Yes."

"Nope. I don't dance with beginners."

These were all moments of incivility, and some were more hurtful, and more anxiety producing, than others. But discourtesy on the dance floor, I learned, was, like anxiety, a fact of life. You had to learn to live with it, to roll with it, to pay it no attention. Most often the shape of dance-floor discourtesy was subtle, like the partner who neither looks at you, smiles, nor speaks, or the partner who drops you cold at the end of a dance as if you were yesterday's garbage.

But the dance floor is like that. It's a place where society's norms are suspended: a place with its own form of etiquette where complete strangers are allowed and encouraged to touch each other, their embrace excused by the power of music. People behave wonderfully under the circumstances. They also behave badly. And I'd grow accustomed to both as I returned, again and again, to the social dance.

To facilitate the journey, Coco one evening explained to me her rules of dance-floor etiquette. They were for me, in terms of my recovery, a quasi–twelve step program, consisting, however, of seven steps for one anxious, would-be ballroom dancer.

Step 1: "Regarding offering, accepting, and declining invitations to dance: It is perfectly acceptable in our community to ask someone to dance whom you don't know, just as it's perfectly acceptable for ladies to ask gentlemen to dance (and from what I hear, the guys like it)."

Step 2: "It's a nice thing to introduce yourself to your partner. A lot of people dance and never exchange names. I think it's polite to say, 'Hi, my name's Coco.'"

Step 3: "If you decline an offer to dance, I consider it impolite just to say no. Offer a legitimate excuse, like, 'Thanks, but I'm a bit tired.' But if you say, 'No, I'm sitting this one out,' and then you proceed to dance with someone else, that's bad manners, too."

Step 4: "It's rude to speak to another person during the course of a dance and ask them to dance the next one. That's called thinking ahead to the next person. I'm there for my partner when I'm dancing with him, and I want him to be there for me."

Step 5: "This is so obvious that you'd think it should be unspoken, but at the end of a dance you should always say 'thank you' to your partner. Only at that point can you move away and find another partner."

Step 6: "What if you go to a dance with a date? It's

common practice, after you arrive, to dance the first dance with your escort. It's also polite to dance the last dance with him or her. And it's probably a good idea to dance a few dances in between (if you want to see them again!). But it's not a good idea to dance every dance with your date. Only beginners do that, and they don't know better."

Step 7: "How close should you hold your partner? 'When you go to the dance, don't dance too close—always make room for the Holy Ghost!' That's what some people say. But really, it depends on the kind of dance you're doing, and on how well the partners know each other. Generally, you don't want your arms to be fully extended. In the ballroom position your elbows need to be bent so there's a circle of space between the two of you. There really should not be much body contact. Unless it's your sweetie you're dancing with."

In the months following my first visit to Cherry Hill, Coco and I went Cajun dancing at least once a week. I grew more and more fluent each time, and the halting nature of my dance-floor demeanor began to give way to assurance and to some sense of ease. I was, in effect, dancing in sentences now, whereas before I had moved about in disjointed words and occasional phrases. My brain was adjusting to planning ahead, to mapping out a dance-floor routine where one move would follow another more or less evenly. No longer was I mostly bobbing up and down, as if stuck in a stutter, with the Cajun jig. Instead, a certain choreography set in:

First bring the lady into a cuddle. From there swing her out to the open position, then back again to a side-by-side turn. Back to a swing out, then right-side pass. Into the cuddle again, first on the right hip, then on the left hip, then back on the right. Back to a swing out and into the skater's position. Cross-armed now, whirl her around in a windmill. And maybe shift down to a little window, and nod to your lady right through the glass.

I was speaking a new language now, thinking somewhat less about what I was doing, and somewhat more about having fun.

As my confidence developed, I began to ask women, strange women, to dance. My register of partners grew. And so did my need for an etiquette counselor. Coco's seven-step program was fine as far as it went. But it didn't address the nuances of close dance-floor combat.

Here is just some of what I encountered:

Imagine embracing, physically embracing, dozens of women—or, if you're a lady, dozens of men—none of whom you've ever met before. There they are, stuck in your arms like a bag of potatoes or a dream come true, depending on your disposition, their faces inches from yours, their bodies brushing your torso, their breath as fresh or as foul as the last beer or breath mint allowed. And you, if you're the guy, are trying to take control, leading your lady with some sense of grace around a crowded dance floor; and you, if you're the lady, are struggling to follow whatever the guy in your arms commands—yes, commands—you to do.

"Wait a minute," thinks the guy. "This woman isn't taking my lead."

"Hold on there," thinks the gal. "This jerk is holding me too tightly and pushing me around as if I were a mop."

Then there are the subtleties: Where do you put your eyes? What do you do with your fingers? What if the lady has really large breasts: should you avoid them or enjoy them? What if the guy is hairy and sweaty and it's summertime and all he's got on is a slinky, slimy tank top: do you really have to touch his bare flesh?

What if the lady is really great looking? And what if she really is not? What if your date is dancing with another guy and smiling like she never smiles when she's stuck on the dance floor waltzing with you?

My first confrontations with issues of etiquette generated mixed results.

Sometimes I behaved admirably, like the time I crushed my partner's toe: "Shit!" she cried, in genuine pain. I was wearing hard-soled shoes; she was wearing soft jazz slippers. I did what I thought was the right thing to do: I stopped the dance to be sure she could walk. Having determined she could, I led her to a nearby seat, bowed as a gesture of contrition, and proffered a sincere apology. And I bought her an orange juice as a token of thanks for putting up with my clumsiness.

Sometimes I was flustered. At Tornado Alley one Friday night, Filé, a Louisiana band, was onstage. They opened a set with "Jolie Blonde," the classic Cajun waltz. A tall brunette, whom I'd seen around, approached me and asked me to dance. I agreed, and off we went. That's when the problem set in. Direct eye contact. She wouldn't take her eyes off mine. For five endless minutes she gazed relentlessly at me. Eyeball-to-eyeball assault in the first degree. This woman never blinked. And to make matters worse, she smiled. Gawked and smiled, as if I were the best little peach she had ever plucked off a tree.

You would think this would have pleased me, for it was, after all, quite flattering. But instead I felt uncomfortable, as if I were being stalked. I squirmed in her arms like a colicky baby, and mostly avoided her eyes by averting mine, as if the act of avoidance would make her go away. I looked at the floor. I looked at the ceiling. I looked at other dancers. I glanced at my watch. Anything to dim that pair of brown headlights beaming in my face.

Finally the music ended, and I thanked her for the dance.

"Why didn't you look at me?" she asked.

She had noticed.

"Huh?" I replied, jolted by the directness of her inquiry.

"You know, we could have had a much more enjoyable experience if you had looked me in the eye while we were dancing."

"Oh," I mumbled, honestly uncertain what to do or say. "Sorry," I added. I turned around and fled to the other side of the club, never to dance with her again.

An incident like that was puzzling, and I still don't quite know what response etiquette demands. But there were more straightforward dance-floor confrontations, where the breach of good behavior was explicit, and the fault all too close at hand. Like the dance I attended with Julie, a longtime platonic pal of mine.

Both of us were unencumbered at the time. She knew that I had started to dance, although I never told her why. One Saturday evening, when each of us was dateless, she asked me to take her out for a Cajun night on the town. We went to the Spanish Ballroom, a wonderful dance hall in Glen Echo Park near Washington, D.C. We got there in time for Coco's workshop, and afterward danced as best we could once the band began to play.

I can't speak to Julie's motives that evening, but I had my agenda: as we waltzed and two-stepped our way around the ballroom, I, to be blunt, was grazing for babes. This, Dr. Gilbert later told me, was a good and healthy thing. A sure sign of my developing recovery, he said. I had been dancing for months, but hadn't dated in two years. Panic disorder dulls the libido. It is difficult to woo a woman when driving to the office is a major life event. But Cajun dancing was beginning to be fun. I was feeling pretty good about my dance-floor self, and slowly but steadily feeling less concerned about my psychiatric disorder. The more I danced, the less I focused on the panic. And the less I obsessed about panic, the more normal my life became, and normalcy, in significant part, included dating women.

Seeking out women was, it turns out, a common dance-floor affectation. Julie was hit on several times that night. And since we were just pals, she didn't mind my roaming eye.

"Hey, Rob, look over there, to your left," she said in the middle of a two-step. "There's my friend Irma [not her real name]. I'll get her to dance with you."

Thus arose the point of etiquette: I didn't want to dance with Irma. I took one look at Irma and thought—I'm ashamed to reveal the truth here—"Well, there's one really ugly woman. I sure as hell don't want to waltz with her."

Out of respect for Julie, who literally threw the unsuspecting Irma into my arms, dance with Irma I did. My grip on her was loose. My posture was off-putting. I didn't speak. I didn't smile. I acted like a jerk.

Six months later, Julie and I went out to dinner. Irma and her boyfriend dropped by. Julie, unbeknownst to me, had invited them along.

"Irma, do you remember Rob?" Julie innocently asked.

"Oh," Irma said. "You're the one who treated me like shit because you didn't want to dance with me."

Like the tall brunette with the fixating eyes, Irma, too, had noticed. I sank into my restaurant seat and flushed with embarrassment and shame. Later on, as I digested the discomfort of that moment, I reconsidered Coco's seven rules of dance-floor etiquette, and I realized that the unstated basis of her etiquette guidebook is the most fundamental rule of all: the ethic of reciprocity, the "golden rule" that underlies, or ought to, all decent human interaction—treat others, on the dance floor or elsewhere, as you would wish to be treated yourself. In the words of the Jewish Talmud: "What is hateful to you, do not do to your neighbor." In the words of the Gospel of Matthew: "All things whatsoever ye would that men should do to you, do ye even so to them."

I doubt that the prophets danced. But they surely had it right. Imagine, I thought, how I would have felt had Irma, informed of my psychiatric problem, dismissed me by saying: "I don't dance with crazies." We all are imperfect, Dr. Gilbert liked to remind me, even the perfectionists among us. And we all wear our imperfections differently. For some, who possess a less than perfect face, the imperfection is apparent. For others, who possess an anxious mind, the fault may be invisible when effectively concealed. In either case the objective, I realized, with respect to etiquette and ethics, is to tolerate the imperfections of others. Stigma is an ugly thing, wherever it appears in life. So is incivility. I vowed never again to discriminate on the basis of looks, or of anything else, on the dance floor.

7

Zydeco

Dialogue with Dr. Steven Gilbert

ME: *So I had been dancing for months, and you know what? I was feeling better. Good enough, I suppose, even to behave badly on the dance floor, just as badly as any normal person would who hadn't coped with panic disorder. In a funny way, that was a nice feeling. It's not that I enjoyed offending a dance partner, because I didn't. But what was nice was the fact that I found myself, day in and day out, focusing on dance, including the etiquette stuff, and I wasn't thinking much at all about anxiety attacks. My mind was constantly wrapped around the ins and outs of social dancing, and this felt good. I felt like I was finally healing.*

DR. GILBERT: *You were healing. Look, the thing with therapy is that it's left-brained. It's an intellectual process in which you talk about something and you get people to think about things. And so much of my training and practice*

*is like that: I talk about feelings with patients.
And talk about them. And talk about them.
And then, over time, the healing somehow takes
place. But there's something missing in that
model. There's something that happens when a
patient gets better. There's some sort of magic
that goes on. And for all the years I've done
this, I'm still sometimes surprised and don't
understand it. I don't know where the magic
happens. But it usually happens off somewhere,
not in here.*

ME: *It happens on the dance floor?*

DR. GILBERT: *For you it was on the dance floor.
Dancing is right-brained. It's art and it's music
and feelings, and you needed all that. And that's
what I mean by magic. You found for yourself a
vehicle that got you from here to there, that got
you to feel better. I think dancing became your
therapy, and Coco became my cotherapist. And
my role at that point was just sort of guiding, or
maybe correcting and adjusting. So I guess what
I'm saying is that I try to create an environment
in which healing can take place, but I don't
provide the healing. The healing comes from
within somebody. And people, like you, find
their own way.*

We all look for markers in our lives: signs, gestures, moments, cues, even little epiphanies that tell us something has changed. Sometimes they come externally, from other people, and the trick is to see them for what they are. When I was a youngster, for instance, wrestling with the eighth-grade challenge of wanting girls to like me, Susan Schneider, the thirteen year old with the biggest set in town, gazed at me and smiled. Thirty-plus years later, I can still see her grin. Her smile was, in a sense, the defining marker of my adolescence, for Susan was really popular, and I knew the instant she singled me out that I could be popular, too. For a shy little kid on the cusp of high school, that was a welcome revelation.

Sometimes, as Dr. Gilbert suggests, the signal comes from within. From a leap that you never believed yourself capable of. As on the day I asked Katie Davis to dance.

It wasn't the dance itself that signaled the fact of my healing. Our encounter lasted just a minute: a few up-and-down gyrations of the Cajun jitterbug, a simple movement called the "cuddle," wherein I spun her counterclockwise, wrapped her in a hug, and drew her to my side.

What mattered instead was the venue—the very public newsroom at NPR; and the woman—whose intellect, good looks, standing, and smile vanquished Susan Schneider's; and the sheer impromptu of the moment—a silly, uninhibited burst of emotion absolutely out of character with anything I had ever done before.

It happened one Sunday morning, in the *All Things Considered* production area. I was the editor of *Weekend ATC,* and Katie Davis was the on-air host.

If Coco had been the primary female figure in my life, Katie was the other woman. I worked with her Wednesdays through Sundays, eight to ten hours a day, each and every week. We knew each other pretty well: our likes and dislikes, our strengths and weaknesses, her passion for dogs, and mine for dance.

While Katie was six years my junior in age, she exceeded me in everything that mattered: brains, beauty, poise, experience, charm, and integrity. Katie, to me, was the perfect colleague. A model of professionalism. A strong soul with a steely will and an understanding heart.

I had, by then, been dancing for four months. My comfort level on the dance floor still required bracing, like trusses to a roof. That would come with seasoning and time. My commitment to the enterprise, however, was steadfast to the point of obsession. I was most decidedly a Cajun dancer—a novice, to be sure—and Katie had been briefed about the nature of my calling.

I had gone dancing the night before, to the Spanish Ballroom at Glen Echo Park. Steve Riley and the Mamou Playboys provided the music. Riley, then barely twenty years old, was a Cajun accordionist and fiddler with a spiky mop of hair and a level of musicianship that far surpassed his age. He had, in fact, been mentored by Dewey Balfa, the great South Louisiana artist, and "Mister Dewey," as Riley called him, had, in young Steve, guaranteed that Cajun music would prosper for some years.

I don't remember how I danced that Saturday evening at Glen Echo. But I do remember having had a pretty good time. The next morning at work, my disposition must have shown it.

"Hey," Katie said, "you're in a good mood. Go dancing again last night?"

"Yep," I replied. "Steve Riley. So when can I edit your piece?"

Someone must have overheard our banter, because minutes later, from the speakers of a nearby CD player in the show director's office, a riff of Cajun accordion music settled over the production area, interrupting a staff meeting on the stories of the day.

Everyone was at the meeting: The producer. The director. The associate producers and production assistants. An engineer. A duty reporter. Plus Katie. And me.

Now, normally this was a serious moment, a time to thrash out our news coverage for the day. What was the lead story? Should we try to get the senator from Texas to comment on pending tax-reform legislation? Whom could we contact in Moscow or Mogadishu to talk about the violence in their streets? As editor, my job was to shape and implement the choices. It was a weighty and sober responsibility, one I was proud to carry, and one I tried to implement with sound judgment, creativity, intelligence, and exacting standards. This was NPR, and there was, in the endeavor, absolutely no room for error.

Instead, that Sunday, in the midst of our morning meeting, I stood up, smiled, and prepared to dance.

The Cajun music was at fault, for it had aroused in me some subliminal trigger. All sense of propriety gave way to pure, unfettered impulse. I turned to Katie Davis and offered up my hands.

"Would you like me to show you how to Cajun dance?" I asked. "Come on. Follow me."

Without awaiting a reply, I grabbed a startled Katie in an open-arm position and led her in a jitterbug all around the room. We looked like a couple of kangaroos.

Katie seemed tense at first, and, she acknowledged later, a little bit embarrassed. But eventually, and gallantly, she warmed up to the task. We gyrated up and then down and then up, first at arm's length, and then in a cuddle, cutting a swath between reels of tape and disheveled remains of the *New York Times* that littered the production area like dust bunnies. As we proceeded, our entire crew—producer, director, and everyone else—just sat there, transfixed, between a flabbergast and flummox.

They applauded when the music stopped, and I bowed to Katie and thanked her for the dance. She didn't, of course, understand what had happened, for she had no inkling of what I had gone through to get me to that moment. But I grasped the meaning as soon as it transpired. Never before had I acted so impetuously, in such a public setting, without regard to how I looked. Never before had I shunted aside my shell of self-consciousness and fear of indignity or degradation. In the most unlikely and sober of venues, in the sanctified newsroom of NPR, I had acted silly. With one simple gesture, with one simple run of the Cajun jig, I, the perfectionist journalist and scholar, had risked a little imperfection, all in the name of some fun. Somehow, in the belly of my workplace, in a Katie Davis cuddle, the serious man who was me embraced a bit of whimsy. And in so doing, I realized that dancing had started to yield some serious dividends, that my panic disorder had finally eased up, and that I was actually, irrevocably, on the mend.

That summer, at Coco's suggestion, I attended a workshop that she had helped to organize. It was held for four days in rural West Virginia at a camp called Buffalo Gap. The place had a huge, wooden open-air dance floor that sat like a jewel in a field of grass, surrounded by green-covered mountains on all sides. If God were a dancer, surely he would go there.

I arrived at Buffalo Gap on a Thursday afternoon. Once I had checked in at the welcome tent—Coco was there working the registration table—I walked up a hill, sleeping bag in tow, toward a cluster of well-weathered cabins. The buildings had planked shoulders that sagged from age, and transparent, rusty meshed screen windows for eyes. They were, nonetheless, still thought to be habitable, stable enough to house the hundred or so dancers who would be in residence.

At the top of the hill, on one of the cabin's rickety porches, a small crowd had gathered around a tall black man in a cowboy hat. He was dancing animatedly with a white woman whose long brown hair fluttered out like streamers as she twirled. An accordionist, also African American, sat on a stool nearby, pumping out a lively tune.

The music resembled Cajun, but had more verve. The rhythms seemed quicker and choppier, jumping around the melody line like grasshoppers rushing down a road. And under it all was a hint of blues—not so much as to slow the tune, for the music had undeniable power and drive, and its voice was cheerful, not sad, but enough to insinuate, most subtly, that this music had paid its dues.

The man in the cowboy hat, J. C. Gallow of Lawtell, Louisiana, was tall and thin and wore jeans and pointy leather boots. The woman in his arms, Millie Ortego, from Opelousas, was petite, but followed his lead with her own sense of strength and dignity. They moved in the closed position, with minimal distance between them. What they were doing did not resemble anything I had ever seen in Cajun dancing. There was no up-and-down jitterbug gyration here, no fancy arm moves. Nor was there the plodding forward motion and regularity of the Cajun two-step. The couple instead shifted smoothly in place, bent-kneed, slightly left then slightly right, their choreography punched with artful hesitations and quick, delicious turns. This was a dance that stood its ground, a dance of self-contained energy and speed. The man at the helm was smiling, taking full stock of the moment. The woman he danced with was smiling, too, mesmerized. Such was the nature of zydeco.

I was stunned by the performance, which struck me as graceful and offbeat and absolutely cool. I wanted to learn this dance, and to learn it well.

For most of the next four days, I steeped myself in zydeco. J.C. and Millie offered intensive beginning workshops each morning and afternoon, and it was at those venues that I and many of the other Washington-area dancers in attendance tried to grasp the basic eight-count pattern of the dance: the SLOW-pause-quick-quick ONE-two-three-four LEFT-right-right-left FIVE-six-seven-eight syntax. It was difficult going for most of us, and certainly for me, because the pauses seemed counterintuitive and tended to trip up the feet.

In the evenings, a zydeco band performed, giving us all the chance to practice what we had learned. Coco had an easy time of it, for she had in fact studied the dance the year before and had fine-tuned her skills with a teaching partner named Ben Pagac. Ben had joined her at Buffalo Gap, and the two of them danced brilliantly, rushing through the eight-count with proficiency and ease, as if SLOW-pause-quick-quick was the normal means of human ambulation.

For me, however, it was a struggle, and it made my head ache, for the music was fast paced, and my brain, which was mired not in anxiety but in a tangle of SLOW-pause-quick-quicks, had trouble keeping up. I was conspicuously self-conscious as I stammered around on the dance floor, but I didn't let that stop me, for most of the others were stammering, too. There were many beginners to dance with that evening, so imperfection ruled the night, and embarrassment was shared.

Oh, but the music. There was nothing imperfect about that. It was eight-cylinder high-five music, bright, bluesy, joyous, and absolutely spellbinding. Propelled by the accordion, and anchored by the repetitious whiskings of a metal rubboard, the music had a force and pleasing agitation that built up steam and would not stop. It was, it seemed to me, pulsing with narcotics. The stuff of serious addiction.

> *Watch that dog—arf arf!*
> *Watch that dog—arf arf!*
> *That dog is mad—arf arf!*
> *That dog gonna bite you—arf arf!*

The lyrics that night were mostly simple and spare, for zydeco was dancing music, not the stuff of ballads. But the words, nonetheless, possessed an aphoristic quality, a hard-life prairie wisdom that went down well with dancing feet:

> *Oh, woman, you know that I loved you a long time ago,*
> *But then you left me for another man,*
> *And now your love has gone sour:*
> *You see that I am doin' fine—*
> *You gonna step into my life?*
> *Oh, please go back where you been,*
> *You know that I don't love you anymore.*

The words were sung by the bandleader, who happened to be the accordionist who had earlier played on the cabin porch. His name was John Delafose, from Eunice, Louisiana, a small prairie town and provincial seat of what some have called "the kingdom of zydeco."

Michael Tisserand, a New Orleans–based journalist, has written a book by that title.[1] It is the principal study of zydeco music.

"The origins of dance, like the origins of music, are always the most elusive of things," Tisserand told me. "Zydeco dancing does not have a recorded history. It is recorded in the bodies of the people who live in South Louisiana. And you can't do an autopsy."

The people he speaks of are men like John Delafose, the Francophone black Creoles who have lived in the region for more than two hundred years. As Tisserand writes in his book:

> In Southwest Louisiana, it is not unusual to hear someone describe himself as both an African-American

---

1. Michael Tisserand, *The Kingdom of Zydeco* (New York: Arcade, 1998).

and a true Frenchman. Creoles acknowledge—indeed celebrate—such a mixed ancestry. Among their forebears are slaves brought directly from Africa, as well as through Haiti and other Caribbean islands. They arrived to discover a rural society that included free blacks who had established themselves long before the Civil War. The character of the state's African-American population changed again after 1791, when *gens libres de couleur*—free persons of color—moved here following the Haitian revolution. The heritage of modern Creoles is a blending of these diverse black groups, as well as American Indians and Europeans, especially French and Spanish. Zydeco, with its mix of European- and African-Caribbean–derived song traditions, is the musical voice of this experience.[2]

Tisserand surmises that African dance traditions— with their "polyrhythmic move your body every which way" quality—had a lot to do with shaping the basic foundation of zydeco dancing. Besides that, he says, the dance developed willy-nilly, without design, in the hearts and minds and legs of the people who maneuvered to the music.

"I don't get a sense that there was a real structure to what was going on," he said. "It had a lot to do with individual expression."

Tisserand recalled in this regard the observation of zydeco artist C. J. Chenier, whose father, the late Clifton Chenier, is considered an icon of zydeco music.

"C.J. said that in the early form of zydeco dancing, everybody just went to boogie," Tisserand noted. "The shoes came flying off, shirts came flying off, sweat was

2. Ibid., 2.

flying, people were sliding across the floor, hopping, skipping, jumping, doing whatever they felt like doing, you know? And that all fit in with zydeco."

Well before Clifton Chenier started out in the 1940s and 1950s, the primary venue for zydeco was the Saturday-night house dance. The Creole house dance was a gathering of family, friends, and musicians, a place where young mannered men would invite a lady to dance by holding out a handkerchief. The club scene eventually took over, and the dance began to change. Today, zydeco dancing has flourishes of hip-hop.

I fell in love with zydeco. It was sweaty, cathartic, and fast-paced dancing, one hundred–mile-per-hour dancing. It made me smile. All the time. Zydeco guaranteed good mental health, and it expedited my recovery. If Cajun dancing maimed my affliction with panic disorder, zydeco would pretty much kill it for good.

Zydeco bands appeared regularly in the Washington, D.C., area after the workshop at Buffalo Gap. J. C. Gallow brought an ensemble to Cherry Hill. John Delafose came, too, playing a gig at Tornado Alley. The Wheaton, Maryland, blues club became a popular port of disembarkation for touring Creole musicians, and eventually for me, the next best thing to Dr. Gilbert's office. Among the accordionists who played there were South Louisiana's finest: Roy Carrier, Lynn August, Rockin' Doopsie, Willis Prudhomme, Jeffrey Broussard, and Boozoo Chavis.

My first visits to Tornado Alley were tentative affairs. I mostly observed from the fringe, because for all my infatuation with zydeco music, I still couldn't handle the dance. It was more nuanced than Cajun, whose steps were straightforward and rhythms quite manageable. I had confidence, even backbone, while Cajun dancing, and enjoyed approaching a range of partners. But zydeco was just plain hard. Despite the Buffalo Gap workshop, I was still a rank beginner, just as I had once been with Cajun dance. And as a rank beginner, I felt, again, inadequate, fearful of publicly revealing my shortcomings. So I did what I had done many months before: I enlisted the help of Coco Glass.

Coco and I had maintained our weekly ritual of private Cajun dance sessions at her apartment. But after Buffalo Gap, and at my insistence, we shifted our focus to zydeco.

At the time, Coco was seeing a lot of Ben Pagac. The two of them taught an hour-long workshop before each Tornado Alley event. Ben was an amazing dancer, whose attention to detail was so pristine that he'd actually done field research in southwestern Louisiana's Creole zydeco clubs. Ben, in short, was Mr. Zydeco.

On my trips to Tornado Alley I'd spend hours observing his dance-floor behavior, the way he engaged his partners, his seamless transitions from move to move. Ben juts his shoulders. I've got to do that. Ben bows his knee. I've got to do that, too. Every ornamentation, every frill, every affectation—if Ben was its author, I would buy the book.

His dances with Coco were especially appealing to watch, for the two of them moved with authority and grace, riding the music as if on horseback, rhythmically cantering to its gait. They had a real dance-floor presence—the Cadillac of dancers—and sometimes the crowds around them would part to give them space to shine.

Ben was mostly restrained in his style, for authentic Creole zydeco was tight and well contained, and he was intent on mirroring the real thing. But on occasion he'd drop in some unexpected gesture or flashy punctuation, and that would make his dancing soar. One of my favorite maneuvers was called the "Phillippe," wherein he and Coco joined at the hips and, in synchronous fashion, tapped out the ONE-two-three-four FIVE-six rhythm with their feet. The move would then end suddenly and spectacularly on the seven- and eight-counts, with a tandem leap backward into a rock step. Ben and Coco looked like a couple of galloping stallions whenever they performed the Phillippe.

Ben was, above all, a relaxed and smooth performer. Panic-free, one might say. His posture was proud but unfettered, like a flag that ripples in the wind. There was a liquidity to his dancing, as shoulders, elbows, knees, head, hips, toes, and fingers flowed in separate currents through a stream of free expression.

I, on the other hand, looked like a stiff. Many

months later, after I got to know him, Ben would tell me that my zydeco dancing in those early days was "mechanical," "jerky," and "marionette-like." "You were so serious and intense on the dance floor," he said. "There was tension in your shoulders and upper body. You just weren't letting loose." It was an assessment that Coco shared, and she resolved to fix it.

She planned an intervention, and retained Ben as her agent-in-chief. "Coco made a point of telling me that I needed to figure out some way to get you to loosen up," he said. "That was my mission."

It happened at Coco's apartment, at one of our regular sessions.

"Ben's coming over tonight," she declared. "He's going to work with us on your dancing. I want him to teach you how to turn."

The zydeco turn. I had seen Ben do it many times, and coveted the move. The zydeco turn is a signature step, a smooth and flashy pirouette that is rendered this way:

From the basic ballroom stance, from the open position, the man and woman disengage, connected by his left and her right hand. They face each other, limbs attached, two arms' lengths apart, and tap out a parallel zydeco step in mirror-image fashion. Then, at the onset of an eight-count musical phrase, and without apparent warning, the man—the woman can do this, too, if she so chooses—breaks away and whips around, affecting the actual turn. At the end of the rotation, the man reconnects with his partner, grabs her again by the hand, and rock-steps backward exactly on the seven-eight. When done properly, the choreography is brilliant. It brightens up the dance like italic lettering, and conveys a bearing that is anything but stiff.

I had never formally met Ben before that evening at Coco's apartment, and the news of his impending arrival set me on edge. In a realm where one's worth is defined by the richness of your dance-floor skills, Ben was a lord and I was a serf, a simple, common beginning dancer. I had never breached protocol to muster the nerve to approach him. He could dance well. I could not. We simply sat at different tables.

Ben was lean and muscular, with exceedingly good looks that gave his dancing extra flair. His face was well chiseled, with a Clint Eastwood ruggedness that was tempered by a Robert Redford glint of sensitivity. The ladies loved him. And I envied all he stood for, for he was the perfect dance-floor personality, and a model, therefore, for emulation. Smooth, relaxed, handsome, poised, stylish, gallant, cool. That was Ben, and I very much wanted to be like him. And I wanted him to like me.

Our meeting at Coco's lasted nearly two hours. It took me that long to learn how to turn.

It wasn't enough for Ben to display, in some superficial manner, just how to execute the zydeco turn. I think he would have liked to have left it at that: two or three demos. Voilà. There you have it. See ya later.

Instead, I demanded—and obtained—a full-fledged seminar. Graduate-Level Zydeco: The Eight-Point Turn—Architecture and Meaning. I prodded Ben. I pushed him. I cajoled and I inquired. Every inch of motion had to be explained. Every step. Every twist. Every pivot. Every pause. All in the name of precious knowledge. All in a search for the perfect turn:

"Now, Ben, on the second beat, does your right leg stomp the floor or just sort of brush against it?"

"Ben, at the three-count, should your shoulders already be at a forty-five-degree angle from your point of departure?"

"Should you, Ben, be completely turned around by the four-count? Or is it better to finish the turn on five?"

"And what should you do with your arms while you're turning?"

"It wasn't easy going," Ben remarked later. "It's not that I was getting to the point of annoyance, but it was an intense session because of your persistence in wanting to get it exact, wanting to know which foot goes here on this count, which foot goes here on that. I was pretty fatigued afterward."

And I was exhilarated. Because after two hours of painstaking instruction, I had grasped the zydeco turn. I knew its molecular structure. I had felt its genetic fingerprint. I understood its heart and soul. Suddenly, I really believed that I could, with time and practice, learn to dance like Ben.

The session with Ben empowered me, and my

zydeco dancing quickly took off. From that point forward I viewed myself as Pagac's disciple and vowed, on the dance floor, to make him proud. I unleashed a holy zydeco crusade, assaulting the space at Tornado Alley with increasing regularity. Whereas before I'd hesitate to step on the floor of a zydeco dance, now I'd seize the moment. Armed with the zydeco turn, my dancing grew hale and bold. Any woman was susceptible to my approach. Skilled. Good looking. Experienced. Savvy. It didn't matter anymore. If she had come to zydeco, I would invite her to dance.

The offensive produced results. Brenda—not her real name—was one of a handful of Tornado Alley zydeco stars: a leading lady whose stunning looks and equally striking dance-floor expertise gave her top-gun social status. Ben could dance with Brenda, and Brenda loved to dance with Ben. But Brenda was off-limits. At least for a novice like me. She may have known that I existed, but she surely paid me no attention. At least not until I asked her to dance.

Midway through our first encounter, I flashed her my zydeco turn.

"You dance pretty well," she said afterward. "What's your name? I need to remember it now."

The irony of this transformation—a point that Coco understood—was the manner in which I achieved it.

"You are very, very analytical," she said of our session with Ben. "It's great that you learned how to turn. But don't forget it's supposed to be fun."

Her point was well taken, for I had, in effect, mastered the turn by attrition, browbeating it out of my teacher. And in my single-mindedness, I had lost sight of the original intent of Ben and Coco's mission—and of Dr. Gilbert's therapy: the need for me to loosen up, to draw in some air, to relax and breathe.

"You still move kinda stiffly, sweetie, even with your turn," Coco teased. "But, God bless you, you do seem to be having a pretty good time."

Stiffly or not, I *was* having fun. With the assistance of Coco and Ben, and through the power of a turn, the dance floor became my playground, a romper room of music and movement where zydeco defined the game. Bit by bit, like an engine charging up with power, the pace of my life quickened, and its quality improved. Things were in place for the next big breakthrough, in which Robert Rand, the serious journalist and scholar, became a skirt-chasing, hard-playing dance-floor stud.

8
Chasing Skirts

My life stopped when I lost you. Then I had a good time.
Michael Doucet, quoting lyrics from a Cajun song

Oh, what a potent elixir zydeco proved to be: a libidinous nectar, sipped with dogged and scrumptious regularity in the second year of my life on the dance floor. No one man in twelve fine months had ever before reaped such sweet rewards: Terry, Amy, Candace, Lynn: well met in the ballroom. Kathleen, Lisa, Carol, Stephanie: swept up with an intoxicating potion of a rubboard and accordion. Jenny, Jacqui, Julie, Anne, Rebecca, Eva, Cindy: lovely women, fourteen-carat women, each engaged by the formerly panicky scholar-journalist-turned-inside-out. Zydeco had claimed me, and I had claimed its battleground: the gridiron of social dance, where anxiety was vanquished, where boys met girls and girls met boys and—rah, rah, sis boom bah—lust quivered, romance exhorted, and hearts pitter-pattered from the scent of possibility.

The transformation in my demeanor, of course, was long in the making, facilitated by ongoing therapy, reflection, introspection, and dance instruction from Coco Glass, with an able assist by Ben Pagac. But once things fell into place, once the dialectic of panic and perfection had materialized into wild dance-floor exultation, I simply could not contain the results. It was as if puberty had struck again: oiled and greased with dance-floor skills and a healthy dose of cockiness, I set out, with adolescent intensity, to have myself one heck of a time. I was the new Mr. Zydeco—at least that's how I viewed it—a sensual dancing machine for whom every woman at each and every dance became potential fodder.

So I dated other dancers. Lots of them.

As noted earlier, I had not gone out with the ladies much during my panic-disordered years. I could barely keep company with myself, let alone with women. The illness was a form of mental impotence. You cannot build a home without a foundation; and for me, dancing, especially zydeco, represented the concrete and girders of reawakened mental health. So my interest in courting females, and the enthusiasm I brought to that pursuit on the dance floor, was, in a way, the surest sign yet of my continuing recovery.

"Hi. You look great out there on the dance floor. Could I have the next dance?"

That was my typical opening line. It was a well-tested, calculated salutation, directed to whoever seemed to catch my eye on any particular evening. The tone of delivery was soft and friendly, punctuated with a smile and an impishly arched eyebrow. The complimentary element of the invitation was lethal: dancers love to be flattered, to have their dancing praised. My target, thus extolled, would think that I oozed with charm. The next dance would always be mine.

"My name is Rob. What's yours?"

Basic courtesy, exchanging names. But ballroom encounters can be fleeting, and dancers often cling to anonymity. Tell them your name and ask them theirs—that shows civility, class, and interest. The golden rule.

"Shall we dance over there, at the foot of the stage?"

A bold move, laced with confidence, for only the best dancers stake out terrain near the band. This will impress her, for sure, for she'll know that her partner is experienced and certain to hold his own. No amateur here, my friend. You've got yourself a guy who can dance.

Once the music begins, the real courtship unfolds, presented in a choreography of steps designed to probe, captivate, please, and beguile. This is the silent, concupiscent side of social dance, the dance-floor seduction.

Step one: I hold my partner reverentially but firmly, as a parent would a newborn. The effect conveyed is calm, contentment: You'll be safe here in my arms.

Step two: I lead with confidence and unfailing precision, further enhancing the mood. By now, if things have gone well, my partner has meshed with my style. She's buckled in and enjoying the ride.

Step three: I show her my open zydeco turn, a gesture of flamboyance—like a peacock flaunting his plumage—designed to astonish and to impress. If she fails to respond, it ends there. She's probably not for me. But if she smiles, or, better yet, if she answers with a turn of her own, I move on fully to engage.

Step four: I draw her a little bit closer as the music picks up speed and the rhythm of the moment wraps around us. She doesn't seem to mind.

"Is this okay?" I ask.

It's best to inquire, just to be certain. Again, the golden rule. The last thing you want to do is cross a line and give offense. Courtesy is the most powerful of dance-floor partners.

Step five: The dance ends, but my embrace, like a postscript, lingers on for a moment. Once I break it, our hands stay clasped and our fingers intertwined.

"Would you like to do another?"

With that I've revealed my true intentions. One dance signals nothing. Two in a row is a virtual relationship.

We zydeco a second time, and maybe a third or fourth. There's a quality, a feeling, about the way we move together—the way we turn—that makes this something special. We laugh amidst the whir of the dance. We look into each other's eyes.

"You're a terrific dancer!" I enthuse. *"You must have danced down in Louisiana!"*

She blushes and smiles. We talk at the break.

"Would you like to get together off the dance floor sometime?" I ask.

"Sure," she says.

We exchange home and work phone numbers. I call her the next evening. We go out for dinner. I call her again. A second date. A third. Then, invariably, one way or another, it ends, collapses, with a big-time thud. Irreconcilable differences with the love of your life. Get to know your dance-floor honey, and wouldn't you know, you have nothing in common. Except for bruised feelings and irritated egos.

"Sure glad I won't have to see her again."

Except that I will, at the very next dance.

To avoid entirely that dilemma, and the awkwardness it entails—among social dancers, there is a consensus that it sucks to see your former sweetheart sway ecstatically in the arms of a new partner—some dance-floor regulars, the more disciplined ones, simply avoid dating other dancers. They engage instead in forms of inconsequential, prophylactic, flirtatious dance-floor behavior. It is a relatively cheerful way of reaping the prurient benefits of serious male-female contact without the subsequent emotional upheaval or, God forgive, the commitment. Anthropologists might call this process interspecies socialization. I like to call it sex on the dance floor.

It comes in different stripes and colors. In its most benign configuration, dance-floor sex is a private affair, conducted consensually in the ballroom by a dancing couple: thighs may brush, cheeks may touch, hips may lock, all in the name of good, clean, hedonistic fun. Sometimes benign dance-floor sex happens between partners who are friends. Sometimes it transpires between strangers. It can be a striking, if short-lived, experience.

I was entirely unprepared the first time it happened to me. I was zydeco dancing with a woman I had never met before. She was, as they say, into me, and I was attracted to her, and we both were into zydeco. My partner had a lovely figure, which she offered up without constraint. Her bosom was profound, and as she jiggled to the music, so did her breasts, which lapped up against my torso with the warmth and inviting allure of waves upon a beach. It was better than Hawaii.

Consensual, flirtatious dance-floor touching is fairly innocuous behavior, when conducted between two interested adults. But sex on the dance floor, in its harshest and most extreme form, can be ugly: a guy overwhelms an unwilling partner with his strength and slams her against him like a piece of meat on a butcher's slab. This form of nonconsensual touching is not only offensive, but borders on assault and battery.

Somewhere between these two extremes lies a double R–rated mode of dance-floor shenanigans, one that I eschew, which involves self-indulgent, provocative, salacious exhibitionism. Groin to groin, with Kamasutra ingenuity as far as positioning goes, a man and woman of this ilk interlock and ride the music as if it were a water bed, humping and moaning and sweating and all but exchanging bodily fluids in the vertical position. As far as I am concerned, only the freest of spirits or most intoxicated of dancers engage in such conduct.

At the zydeco dances in Washington, D.C., one couple stood out in this regard. They shall remain nameless here. Crowds would watch them with a mix of voyeuristic fascination and puritanical mortification. Each of them was a professional, with impressive affiliations. Each was middle-aged, and often came scantily clad — he in a loose-fitting open shirt, she in a miniskirt with Band-Aids for panties that showed when she twirled. At its most sublime, their routine was alluringly poetic: seductive hips and undulating shoulders woven together to evoke the carnal underbelly of the human experience. But mostly they just grinded, wagging their genitals without regard to local community standards.

"I call it sleaze-and-slime dancing," said Stan Fowler, dance director at the Spanish Ballroom in Glen Echo Park near Washington, D.C., a venue for many zydeco dances. During the nineties, Fowler oversaw thousands of dances at Glen Echo, patrolling the ballroom in signature khaki shorts and an olive green shirt for the U.S. Park Service, which runs the facility. "They call me a dance ranger," he said. His analytical skills with regard to dance-floor behavior would impress Dr. Gilbert.

"When a really nice-looking lady shows up, you've got what I call the sharks and the porpoises," he said. Sharks are the skirt-chasers, "the guys who are looking for meat," the guys who want to score. "Porpoises are just looking for someone to play with," a beach ball "to bounce around for a while," a "good playmate" to engage for the duration of a tune and then to part with once the dance is over.

A social dance attracts these and other species for good psychological reasons, according to Fowler. "A dance serves as a reservoir of keeping people mentally or physically comfortable with the stuff they need," he said, "with the stuff they could get in a marriage if they had one. You know, those attraction highs. You dance with somebody and you go, 'Wow, this person was wonderful!' You've looked into their eyes and you go, 'Yeah, this was great!' And then the next person you dance with you have the same thing, and you've just wiped the other one right out. So it goes, through the whole night. And you leave and you go, 'This was nice.'"

Fowler, himself a veteran social dancer, acknowledged that overtly sexual antics on the dance floor offend many dancers. "What's a ripe banana to one person is a rotten banana to another," Fowler drolly observed. "My boss once said about a couple of dancers: 'I don't even let my husband get that close to me!'"

Like it or not, be it zydeco or Cajun or other forms of social dance, the hint of romance or of sexual possibility is always there. It is as surely a ballroom component as the music is. It is the reason, in days gone by, some conservative communities frowned on social dance. It is the reason, in simpler times in South Louisiana, a male and female zydeco dancer at first introduction would grip one another from opposite ends of a handkerchief, rather than take the risk of flesh touching flesh.

Looking back on it all, the sexual side of Cajun and zydeco dance was, for me, undeniably part of the appeal, and doubtless part of the cure. Human sexuality is part of who we are. At the height of my illness, there was no space in my mind for the opposite sex. As I recovered, things changed. Far better to anticipate a social dance with all its romantic possibilities than to anticipate anxiety. Chasing after women was a pleasurable endeavor, and pleasure, diversion, enjoyment, entertainment, fun, this was the stuff that fueled my return to health.

9
Boozoo

On a Wednesday night at Tornado Alley, in the midst of the merriment that was my second year on the dance floor, a zydeco group called Boozoo Chavis and the Majic Sounds performed onstage. The band had traveled north for the gig from Lake Charles, Louisiana, and their leader, Mr. Wilson Anthony "Boozoo" Chavis, was the senior statesman of South Louisiana Creole music. Next to the late Clifton Chenier, Chavis probably did more than anyone else to propagate the modern zydeco sound. Ask him and his supporters who the king of Louisiana zydeco is, and the retort "Boozoo, that's who!" is what you'd get.

It was a work night, but the dance floor was stuffed with zydeco enthusiasts, and the party didn't end until well after one. Not that Boozoo, a spirited gentleman in his sixties, wouldn't have carried on until dawn, had the management allowed:

> Dance all night, stay a little longer,
> Dance all night, stay a little longer,
> Dance all night, stay a little longer,
> Can't see why you can't stay a little longer.
> Take off your shoes, throw 'em in the corner . . .
> Take off your wig, throw it in the corner . . .

Take off your drawers, throw it in the corner . . .
Can't see why you can't stay a little longer!

It was one of Boozoo's signature songs, rendered that night with his characteristic blend of impishness, vigor, bluster, and pride. Boozoo more than played a song, he anthropomorphized it, filling its form with wit and personality. With a voice cast in dust from the road and a boppy, percussive accordion style, Boozoo regaled onstage, energizing dancers with sonorous riffs and simple words that evoked the South Louisiana prairie life he knew best: the times he was so poor that "a paper in my shoe" was the only way to keep his feet warm; a paean to Dog Hill, his Lake Charles home "where the pretty women at"; a tongue-in-cheek tribute to his wife, Leona, who once had a party where "everybody got drunk"; a rollicking zydeco tune to honor Motor Dude, one of his horses.

Of all the zydeco events I attended that year, I remember the Boozoo Chavis show the best. It was, in no small part, because he was Boozoo, and it was a real treat to dance to his music. But mostly the evening stuck in my mind because of what happened beforehand.

"Ben is out of town this week. Would you like to teach the zydeco workshop with me at Tornado Alley?"

Coco's telephone call astonished me. Ben—my role model and indisputably the best zydeco dancer around—was unavailable, and Coco wanted *me* to take his place. She wanted *me* to be *Ben*. At a workshop before a *Boozoo Chavis* performance, no less. I was honored and absolutely thrilled.

"You bet," I said. "When can I come over to prepare?"

We met at Coco's apartment for two consecutive nights before the actual event. The Allied invasion of Normandy could not have been more meticulously thought through. My role was that of the workshop's supporting actor: I was to back up Coco and demonstrate the men's part as she explained, layer by layer, the constituent elements of the zydeco dance. That meant, at the outset, nothing more than standing in front of a row of guys, who'd been separated from the ladies, and guiding them slowly through the slow-pause-quick-quick, left-right-right-left pattern of the zydeco choreography. It was a simple task, but I wanted to get it absolutely right, so we rehearsed the routine until I was certain my teaching style projected the right mix of expertise, insight, and informality.

Then there was the more complicated challenge of teaching the closed position, and getting the partners, thus attached, to move as a unit to the zydeco rhythm.

"First off we'll have them practice giving weight," Coco said. "I'll ask the men and women to couple up—your job will be to ensure that everybody has a partner, okay?—and I'll tell each pair of dancers to face each other, take each other's hands, bend their elbows, and lean backward and away—like opposite ends of a stretched-out rubber band—bending their knees and squatting down as far as they can without toppling over. That's called giving weight. There has to be the right amount of tension, or balance, so that each partner's weight is completely supported. Having the proper balance with your partner is the key to zydeco."

Once that was done, Coco said she would position the couples in a closely held ballroom stance. "They need to be real cozy, 'cuz that's the only way to keep up with the music, so you go around and coax the shy people into snuggling up to their partners, okay?" Once the couples were positioned, Coco said she and I would walk them in tandem through the zydeco steps.

"What about the zydeco turn?" I asked.

"Too complicated for beginners, sweetie. But you can show them what it looks like in the demo."

The demo, Coco explained, would open up the workshop. It was, in effect, a performance, in which she and I would demonstrate, to music, what zydeco dancing looked like for those who had never seen it.

I had, of course, watched demos many times before: Coco would do them at all of her Cajun and zydeco workshops. For those who were new to zydeco, and even for those who were not, the demo, as performed by Coco, was always a joy to watch. It was, in fact, the highlight of the show, like a fireworks finale, except that it came first. She would invariably blow the crowd away. But her partner had always been Ben, and the two of them would put on such a spirited and skilled performance that I had an awfully hard time figuring out how I, Coco's student, could adequately stand in. But what a privilege and an opportunity, I thought, to be Ben's understudy; to be for a moment the real Mr. Zydeco; to dance, literally, in his shoes. And what better way to impress the women, in the midst of my second-year run on the dance floor? And what could be a more appropriate symbolic public act with which to exclaim, at least to myself (for I had told nobody except Dr. Gilbert and Coco about my psychiatric crisis, such was the strength of my fear of stigmatization), that my health was being restored, that I could cut loose and have fun, and that my panic disorder was succumbing to the restorative force of social dance?

We practiced our routine for hours, which tested even Coco's patience. "I want to get the demo right," I insisted. "I want to look really good out there with you on the dance floor."

"Relax, bud," Coco chided. "Don't be so serious. You'll do just fine. Just get out there and enjoy yourself—it's s'posed to be fun, remember?"

Coco selected a song called "Zydeco Extravaganza" as the music for our demo. I had never heard it before, and it struck me as one of the most exciting and dance-able tunes ever written, a cannonade of bouncy, single-row accordion riffs that demanded serious movement. The tune was the brainchild of a group appropriately called Zydeco Force.

The power behind "Zydeco Extravaganza" was its

simplicity: the tune repeated, with occasional embel-
lishments, a single, captivating twelve-note musical
phrase over and over again. The result was an appealing
zydeco mantra that seeped into the brain's gray matter
and triggered whatever it is inside us that mesmerizes,
scintillates, overcomes, and casts a spell. "Zydeco Extravaganza" was enormously popular in South Louisiana, lending its name to a television show—the zydeco
equivalent of *American Bandstand*—and to an annual
music festival.

The lyrics to the song were as sparse as the music
was simple. Again, repetition was the key: the names of
a handful of popular zydeco clubs were chanted once
and then twice and then some more, like hosannas at a
religious revival:

> *Richard's club!*
> *Slim's Y-Ki-Ki!*
> *Papa Paul's in Mamou-oo!*
> *Don't forget the Bamboo-oo!*

Of the four dance establishments mentioned in
the song, the first two—Richard's (pronounced, as in
French, "Ree-shardz") and Slim's—were the most famous. Coco had told me that these were the well-
springs of zydeco music, the Jerusalem and Mecca of
Louisiana Creole dance culture.

"I've never visited them, but Ben has," she said.
"And so should you, if you really want to learn how to
dance."

Up until that point, I had never thought about traveling to Louisiana. For one, there was really no necessity. Louisiana had come to me. There was ample opportunity to dance to genuine Cajun and zydeco bands in the Washington, D.C., area, sometimes as often as two or three times a week. The bands themselves marveled at the presence of the vibrant and loyal Louisiana dance clique in the nation's capital, of all places. They must have considered it odd—especially the black Creole zydeco musicians—that a company of well-educated, highly paid, nearly middle-aged men and women, overwhelmingly white men and women, who worked in and around the federal government, would attach themselves with such unabashed enthusiasm to a people and music and culture and dance that was, after all, on the other side of the racial divide.

That was the other issue. Race. I would have to confront it—my prejudices, fears, ignorance, and preconceptions—if I went to Louisiana. And I never had reason to do that before. My dancing friends and I were white. The zydeco musicians, and most of the clubs they played in back home—including Richard's and Slim's—were black. We certainly considered ourselves to be tolerant regarding issues of race relations. But for me, at least, my views were theoretical and entirely untested. I had been reared and educated in a wholly white environment, in a middle-class white suburban Jewish ghetto near Chicago, a city Martin

Luther King Jr. once described as the most racially divided in the country. My neighbors and relatives called black people *schvartzers*. I had never had any African American friends. And I had certainly never been a lone white man in an all-black dance club. The prospect of visiting South Louisiana for the purpose of zydeco dancing was, therefore, pretty daunting.

But Ben had done it. And so, I'd heard, had a handful of others. It was, to their minds, a pilgrimage, a rite of passage, the very best way to improve their dance-floor skills. Once you had danced in South Louisiana you could rightfully claim you knew how to zydeco. It was, I'd imagined, like traveling to a foreign land in order to pick up the language. Book-learning Russian had never brought me fluency. I obtained that only after studying in Leningrad and living in Moscow. So it must be with the language of zydeco: I would never really learn how to speak it, never really understand its nuances and intonations, until I had danced at Richard's Club and Slim's Y-Ki-Ki. That was the message I took away from the lyrics and rhythms of "Zydeco Extravaganza."

The Tornado Alley dance workshop was scheduled to begin at eight o'clock. The band was to play at nine. Coco and I arrived an hour early. She had dolled up for the occasion, wearing her favorite teaching costume: a short black skirt that twirled when she spun, black tights, black top, a wide black belt, and black leather dance shoes. I had dolled up, too, hoping to strike a relaxed and natty figure in a freshly ironed white oxford-cloth shirt, hot-from-the-dryer raven-black jeans, and white running socks. My shoes were Rockports, their rubber soles worn ideal-for-dancing-flat by a year's worth of Cajun and zydeco activity.

Boozoo Chavis and the Majic Sounds were already there when we walked in. They were seated near the dance floor at wooden booths, eating plates of barbecue. Boozoo was wearing a Stetson hat. Their stage had been set, the sound check completed, and Mr. Chavis, it seemed, with nothing else to do, was settling in to watch the zydeco dance lesson.

At eight o'clock, it began. Coco walked onto the dance floor, welcomed the crowd of fifty or so people who had come for the workshop, introduced me—"This is Rob, my dance and teaching partner"—and directed the man at the sound booth to hit the music. A butterfly flit in my belly. I was pumped, as excited as a kid about to visit Disneyland. It was time for the demo. Show time. Broadway. The Bigs. Inexplicably, amidst the buzz, my mind wandered, and settled, for a beat, on the precipice of panic.

I looked down at my feet and drew a breath. There it was again, my most unwelcome visitor, leaping like a lightning flash from the bottom of my psyche to the forefront of my consciousness.

I considered the option of having a panic attack, after all this time, in front of all these people. But the thought disappeared as quickly as it had materialized.

With that it was over.

Nothing transpired.

I struggled to understand what had happened. This flash of panic, I reasoned, was probably the product of the circumstance: I was feeling anxious out there on the dance floor, about to perform my demo with Coco, and my panic disorder had once thrived on anxiety, stress, and the fear of performing in public imperfectly. But circumstances had changed, and so had I. I had learned from Dr. Gilbert that anxiety can be a healthy response to positive stress. It need not call forth panic. I concluded that what I was sensing was perfectly okay, the normal jitters anyone would feel standing there in Ben Pagac's place, about to dance solo before a crowd.

It was time to zydeco. That is what mattered. That's what I told myself. That's how I regained my focus. It was time to cut loose with the woman who had opened up my world to social dance, time to perform in the club I had come to adore, time to step out, touch, and turn as Boozoo—That's Who!—the icon of my favorite music, sat there, munching barbecue, making ready to honor the night and us with his gift of accordion. I was in reality feeling great, ready to savor the wonderful moment about to transpire. There was no place here for panic disorder, although I wondered, even then, considering my visitor's brief and unexpected call, whether the panic would ever wholly leave the dormant cellar of my mind.

The soundman hit the play button, and the accordion voice of Zydeco Force rolled over the dance floor.

"Owwwweee!" Coco squealed.

We were off.

> *Richard's club!*
> *Slim's Y-Ki-Ki!*
> *Papa Paul's in Mamou-oo!*
> *Don't forget the Bamboo-oo!*

I released, like a whiff of grapeshot, my entire stockpile of moves in that sixty-second demo: rock backs, clockwise twirls, forward steps, backward steps, syncopated toe taps, and, of course, the open-position zydeco turn. I don't know what we actually looked like, dancing there before the crowd. Coco, I'm certain, was grounded and smooth. I may have seemed like a stiff next to her. But in my head, where I processed the experience, I was the coolest, hottest, hippest, most eloquent zydeco dancing man in town. By the time it had ended, Coco was breathless, and the people around us rewarded our performance with oohs and ahs and spirited applause. I tried to contain a smile, but failed. What delicious joy I felt. What pristine, unadulterated glee. This was the high point of my life, or so, at least, it seemed.

The rest of the workshop passed in a blur.

Afterward, Coco told me how delighted she was with the way I had handled the performance. "I was looking at that joyful face of yours while we danced, and I realized how far you had come," she said, as if somehow she knew what had gone through my mind in the moments before the demo. "It gives me great pleasure to know that you love to dance and you understand, as I do, the joy it can bring. We're equals on the dance floor now, sweetie. You've become my dance partner, not my student. I don't have to be your mother hen anymore."

We hugged, and I wandered away. That's when I happened upon Boozoo Chavis, who was lingering at his booth. Boozoo had witnessed the demo and workshop, and as I strolled by, he caught my eye and nodded.

"Man, y'all dance real good up here in D.C.," he said. It was a compliment. Directed at me.

"Thanks, Boozoo," I replied. I grinned, averted my eyes, and floated up to heaven. Where God reached out and touched me on the shoulder.

"It is time to journey to Louisiana," God said. *"Eh toi! Yeah, you right!"*

10
In South Louisiana

On a wind-chilled, sleet-filled Wednesday afternoon the next March, as a diehard winter poked the nation's capital with a jet stream of nasty Canadian air, I packed up my dancing shoes, wished my friends and colleagues well, boarded a plane, and flew south toward springtime: to South Louisiana, where warm, coastal marshlands nestled against an inland gumbo of fresh-water swamps, Spanish moss, bayous, and prairies; and where, it was said, if you listened closely, the evening air, unstained by city sounds, might pulse with the reedy echo of a roadhouse Cajun or Creole accordion, and the night's constellations, blemished only by the imagination, might two-step or zydeco accordingly.

The trip had been put off for months because of logistics: I couldn't find a dance partner.

I wasn't inclined to embark on the journey without one. A partner would act as a safety net, someone to dance with when skilled local women rejected my advances, as surely they would, for I would be a stranger of uncertain ability. And—more to the heart of the matter—I needed a partner to help me maneuver in and around the issue of race: a backup to ease the apprehension—the anxiety—I'd certainly feel as I walked, for the first time in my life, into an all-black environment.

Coco was my first pick as a traveling companion, but she declined the invitation. "Too much to do at work," she said. "Can't get away. Besides, I've met a fella."

I was left without a second choice until I encountered Diana Steele. I had seen Diana at the Boozoo Chavis dance, and at other Cajun and zydeco events around town. I found her to be quite attractive, with long brown hair and sympathetic eyes and curves that would turn any guy's head. And her style was pleasantly offbeat, for she dressed with a touch of down-to-earth, urban funk, a kind of anti-Gap cachet I was too shy to emulate and because of that admired.

And Diana played the fiddle—the Cajun fiddle—and she'd been to Louisiana once before, and knew her way around.

I had first made Diana's acquaintance at the Glen Echo Spanish Ballroom. A zydeco band was performing. We never even danced. We just talked, at length and animatedly, an indication of some mutual interest. I asked her out right then and there. She said in principle she'd love to get together, but was moving the next week to Chicago, where she had gotten a job as a science writer. I told her Chicago was my hometown, and offered to send her some tips on how to survive there. We exchanged mailing addresses, and traded several letters over the next few months. When I broached the idea of dancing together in Louisiana, she accepted enthusiastically, even though we hardly knew each other.

"I wasn't sure what you expected of this trip and of me," she said later. "I wasn't there to be on a date with you. I was there to be with someone who had an appreciation of Cajun and zydeco culture. And who could help me out when I got into trouble."

Our base of operations was to be Lafayette, a once-thriving-turned-under-the-weather oil town that had lost its economic balance when prices for crude nosedived in the 1980s. By the nineties, tourism had joined oil as a major industry, for Lafayette sat at the heart of Cajun country—Acadiana—and the town was a gateway to Cajun and zydeco music and dance.

A first-time visitor to any location is probably taken by the novelty of it all, by sights and sounds that, because of their freshness, taste particularly flavorful. I came to Louisiana with an educated palate, having traveled around quite a bit in my life. Moscow, Athens, Rome, Paris, Jerusalem, Vienna, Munich, Kiev—that's just a partial list of the places I had seen. But Louisiana struck me, a northerner on his first trip to the Deep South, as especially tangy. The scenery was thick and lush and totally exotic. I spent a day as a tourist, taking it all in, before Diana's arrival.

The best way to absorb the lay of the land was by automobile. And the recommended road through South

Louisiana, and to Lafayette, was Interstate 10, which cuts through Cajun country like a shish-kebab skewer.

The journey began in New Orleans, at the western rim of Lake Pontchartrain, a 630-square-mile body of water that kept the state's seafood industry fat with blue crabs and shrimp and trout and flounder. The highway there was flat and buttressed, and flew over the lake at just above sea level, like a stone skipping water. The LaBranch wetlands lay just below, the muddy surface brilliantly flecked with brush strokes of avian white—the snowy egrets at the lake's swampy edge, stalking whatever it is that egrets stalk in the shadow of New Orleans.

One hour later, the approach to Baton Rouge. To the right, a single-digit skyline: the towering walls of the new state capitol. At thirty-four stories it is the tallest repository of state power in the nation.

The structure, I knew, had an interesting history. It was conceived by Louisiana's most famous political native son, Governor, then Senator, Huey P. Long, who in 1935 was shot and killed by an assassin in one of the capitol's corridors.

The midday sun flicked off the building's limestone facade, switching on a childhood memory: *All the King's Men,* the old Hollywood film, with Broderick Crawford as Willie Stark, a fictional character based on Huey Long. I loved this film when I was a kid, and considered it an American classic: a cinematographic etude that totally captured a person, his time, and his place: Huey Long's Louisiana, a state with a dangerous, populous streak and a penchant for corruption.

Until I took up Cajun and zydeco dancing, *All the King's Men* had been my only point of reference to Louisiana.

Interstate 10 turns away from Baton Rouge at the Mississippi River, where a nearly mile-long bridge arcs over the water like a steel rainbow. If you are looking, as I was, to understand Louisiana, the riverbanks below offered as good a take as any:

There was the Port of Greater Baton Rouge, a reminder of the river's link to commerce. There on its banks was the Exxon refinery, as well as other chemical plants, evidence that oil and gas were still major players in the state's economy. There, too, was *The Belle of Baton Rouge,* a riverboat casino, its architecture echoing the Old South, its function revealing the ubiquity of legalized gambling in Louisiana. And there, of course, were the levees, which kept the river in tow.

These man-made embankments of land were, in a sense, a monument to the Mississippi and a sign of respect for the power of its waters. When angered, the waters could bring flooding and misery. When tame, they breathed life into the state, providing a channel of trade and recreation, as well as a link to the past. The bayous and swamps of the state's southern region are attached by geography and history to the Mississippi River, and are part of its alluvial plain. These tributary waters are central to Louisiana's psyche, and were what I always conjured up whenever I heard a plaintive Cajun waltz.

Not long after crossing the Mississippi, Interstate 10 turns directly west toward Lafayette, running over Louisiana's greatest swamp, the Atchafalaya Basin. The basin is fed by the Atchafalaya River, the Mississippi's principal distributary. Some 30 to 50 percent of the Mississippi's waters flow into the Atchafalaya, where they meander south to the Gulf of Mexico.

This stretch of I-10 is known as the Atchafalaya Freeway, and it is one of the most beautiful pieces of interstate highway I had ever seen. The swamp, which is larger than the Everglades, was easily visible from my car. It reached out to the horizon.

The waterscape was broad and stunning, a wilderness of tupelo trees, black willow, and cypress festooned in Spanish moss, which drooped off the branches like mangled, sinewy gray icicles. The scene was a thick tableau of blues and greens and grays and browns, a brilliant menagerie of river otter and egrets and heron and wood ducks, of bald eagles, crawfish, nutria, and alligators. It was the stuff that defined South Louisiana.

Fiddle with the radio as you pass over the swamp, and you'll probably come upon a station playing old-time Cajun music. The bright riffs of the accordion only sharpen the picture around you. It is breathtaking, really; a delicious blend of sound and sight, a moment when the senses stand ramrod straight at attention, etching a memory that will linger the rest of your life. I was pleased I had come to Louisiana. And I couldn't wait to dance.

A half hour later, enter Lafayette.

Diana had arranged for us to stay at the home of John and Barbara Davenport, a Washington-area couple. We would have the place to ourselves. The Davenports had purchased the property for utilitarian reasons: they loved the Cajun two-step, waltz, and jig, and traveled to Lafayette often to dance. The house—a white two-storied building that creaked at its joints from wear and tear—appeared pleasant enough, although it sat in a slightly beleaguered part of town. But everything worked, there was coffee in the cupboard, and the rent was outrageously cheap—ten bucks a night provided you vacuumed and locked up after checking out.

Diana arrived in the evening. We greeted each other with a hug.

This was her second visit to South Louisiana, and she came with a well-thought-out agenda, one that revealed the impressive set of contacts she had culled from her previous trip. She told me her primary mission, besides dancing, was to procure a freshly made violin from Lionel Leleux, Cajun fiddle maker, of Leleux, Louisiana. Lionel was a genuine craftsman, and an artist of some renown. To own a Leleux was to own a Cajun Stradivarius. Diana had also earmarked a day to go horseback riding at the ranch of Geno Delafose, a zydeco bandleader.

She told me she felt a bit like a groupie.

"For me," she said, "it's not the movie stars, it's the musicians. I have to be up close and touch them. I can't adore them from afar. I want to get inside their lives somehow. I want Lionel and Geno to be my friends.

"I think it has to do with my search for cultural identity," she explained. "I'm the quintessential WASP. My relatives came on the *Mayflower.* I don't know where my roots are. When I stumble across people who have a very well-identified culture that is very exuberant in a way that my Puritan ancestry is not, I find that I have a love affair with it. But I'm frustrated that I can never really become it. It is never going to be my cultural ancestry. But I've come pretty close. Having a fiddle made by Lionel Leleux, I feel like I'll be carrying a torch, always."

I told Diana that my agenda differed somewhat from hers. I wanted to spend my days working. I had brought along a microphone and tape recorder, intending to find a Cajun or zydeco dance story to air on *Weekend All Things Considered.* There was, to my mind, no better way than a little bit of journalism to meet the local people and to get a sense of their culture, and maybe to learn some more about dance. So Diana and I agreed to go our separate ways during the daylight hours. We resolved to hook up in the evenings to dance.

We also agreed to sleep in separate rooms. Although, as it happened, by the end of the trip we would become husband and wife.

Marriages develop in all sorts of ways. Some people wed their high school sweethearts. Some wind up with a soul mate or friend. Others give in to wining and dining and the well-planned-out romantic pursuit. Still others succumb, come what may, to sexual combustion and to the draw of the flesh. Whatever its origin, marriage is usually the product of reflection, and carries with it some degree of notice. Our conjugal arrangement, which was struck by necessity, was one of convenience. It came about, at least from my perspective, without premeditation. But that is the nature of shotgun weddings.

The question of matrimony was not on the table when Diana and I went dancing our first night together in South Louisiana. At her suggestion, we dropped in at Mulate's, the Cajun restaurant and dance place a half hour's drive east of Lafayette, in a town called Breaux Bridge. Steve Riley, the wonderfully talented young musician I had once seen in Washington, was performing, along with his group, the Mamou Playboys. As soon as we walked in, half of the band looked up at Diana and nodded or waved in recognition. I was impressed.

It was a Thursday night, and Mulate's was fairly

empty. The handful of couples on the dance floor appeared to be regulars. Diana and I did a waltz and a two-step—a foray that, in my mind at least, established my dancing credentials—and then, at the break, she retired to chat with members of the band. I occupied a chair at the side of the dance floor, surveyed the scene for potential partners, and, when the music started up again, tried to collect the nerve to ask someone to dance.

It was surprisingly difficult to do, and not because of race. Everyone at Mulate's was white. But these folks were authentic Cajun dancers, nursed at the traditional house dance, the *fais do do,* and schooled on "Jolie Blonde." As adults they sashayed with exquisite skill. Coco Glass's lessons notwithstanding, I was an outsider, a Jewish guy from Chicago, a man from the far side of Oz. Hava Nagilah. How could I ever be comfortable at Mulate's?

As I wallowed in such thoughts, a middle-aged woman with dark brown hair marched up and invited me to dance. She was one of the Mulate's regulars, dispatched to make me feel welcome. I smiled and thanked her and held out my hand. We took to the floor and enjoyed a waltz. I completed the dance without a stumble. With my confidence restored, I asked her if she'd like to do the next one, which turned out to be a fast-paced jig. She agreed, but suggested I follow her lead, the better to show me the local style of the dance. So as Steve Riley pumped out notes at a bullet-train tempo, the lady in

my arms drew me through a whipsaw of spins, gyrations, and breakneck turns. I kept up with her fine. It
was lots of fun.

She told me her name was Nelda. I asked Diana
later on if she knew who the woman was.

"Nelda Balfa," she said. "One of Dewey's daughters."

As in Mister Dewey Balfa, the legendary fiddler
who had helped to make Cajun music the centerpiece
of an Acadiana cultural renaissance. It was Dewey Balfa
who, in the fifties, sixties, and seventies, promoted the
South Louisiana fiddle and accordion sound at a time
when many Cajuns, in the name of assimilation, had
discounted their French heritage as embarrassing and
hick. By the eighties, that opinion had changed, thanks
in no small part to the way Dewey Balfa had put his
music out there, and to the way his music made his
people feel. To be a Cajun became a matter of pride,
and Balfa's music fueled that self-esteem as much as
anything.

It was, I figured, serendipity—and no small
honor—to have had Nelda Balfa as a partner for my
first-ever dance with a real Cajun. She had welcomed
me to Mulate's without regard to who I was. It was a
kind gesture that led me to focus my journalistic efforts
onto Cajun dance.

Nelda had told me that one of the very best dance
halls was a nearby Breaux Bridge club called La Poussiere. She suggested I try it out. French-speaking ladies
and gentlemen would be there, she said, real old-timers.

There was no better place to capture the heart of an evening of Cajun music and dance. Two days and some set-up work later, with a microphone and SONY TC-D5M recorder in hand, I visited the club. This story later aired on *Weekend All Things Considered:*

> RR: There is something reassuring about predictability. A sense of security in an old, comfortable-shoe kind of way that derives from the knowledge that there are some aspects of life you can count on to provide comfort food for the soul.
>
> [sounds of the crowd at La Poussiere]
>
> FIRST CAJUN DANCER: Oooh, every Saturday! Walter Mouton been playing about twenty-nine years over here.
>
> RR: For thirty years, actually. On Saturday nights, Walter Mouton has mounted the squat platform stage in this Southwest Louisiana dance parlor and, before a crowd of several hundred neatly dressed young-at-hearts, picked up the accordion and cut loose.
>
> [sound of Cajun accordion music playing gaily]
>
> RR: It's the kind of music, the people say here, that propels you onto the dance floor.
>
> FIRST CAJUN DANCER: It's a smooth, dancin' music. In other words, Walter Mouton, when they make a mistake, every dancer make a mistake.

RR: It's the kind of music the Cajun people of this part of the country take pride in.

Second Cajun Dancer: Well, he's the only musician that plays French music like French music should be played. That's why I come to dance to his music every Saturday night.

[more sound of Cajun accordion music]

RR: *La Poussiere* is the French word for "dust," as in the dust the people here kick up as they fill this cavernous, low-ceilinged place with two-steps and waltzes and, if Walter Mouton moves them just right, an occasional arm-flailing Cajun jitterbug. The couples circle the wooden dance floor in a steady, counterclockwise flow, a mesmerizing current of men in white or plaid shirts and ladies in dresses or slacks, their hair permed up in a bouffant style. It's most definitely a fifty- and sixty-year-old crowd, or even older.

First Cajun Dancer: Oooh, they got a lot of people. There's old people. They come to take exercise over here. You see, if they quit coming over here, they gonna die. They die! You can't stay all the time in a house now, brother. You gotta get out and work!

RR: And work they do, each Saturday night at La Poussiere, from 8:30 to 12:30. For an admission price of two dollars they get exercise, fellowship, and sometimes a free bowl of gumbo. And, of course, with reassuring regularity, the music of Walter Mouton and his band.

[The music plays and ends, followed by enthusiastic applause.]

WALTER MOUTON: My name's Walter Mouton and when you think about Saturday in La Poussiere, you're just thinking about a plain, old-fashioned good time. Good music, good people, and you can't ask for anything more than that.

[sounds of a happy, boisterous crowd]

RR: This is Robert Rand reporting.

The night after dancing at Mulate's, Diana and I planned to visit Richard's Club, the squat prairie roadhouse off Route 190 in Lawtell, forty-five minutes northwest of Lafayette. Richard's, along with Slim's Y-Ki-Ki, was a zydeco dancing institution, a place where the best bands played and the best local dancers danced. It was also, as I well knew, a black club, and a centerpiece of Creole culture.

I looked forward to the excursion with a mixture of apprehension and excitement: excitement, of course, because I loved to zydeco, and this would be my first tour on the music's front lines; and apprehension because I didn't know how I would be treated—and how I would react—as an outsider from a very white world.

The excitement was fueled by the news that Beau Jocque and the Zydeco Hi-Rollers would be playing at Richard's Club that night. Beau Jocque was a zydeco phenomenon, a physically towering hulk of a man whose music, driven by a triple-row accordion, was said, by those who had heard it, to overpower.

The apprehension was eased somewhat by Judith Meriwether and Philip Gould. I had met Judith at KRVS-FM, the NPR member station in Lafayette. And I knew of her husband, Philip, a gifted photographer, through a coffee-table picture book called *Cajun Music and Zydeco*.[1] Barry Jean Ancelet, the University of Louisiana at Lafayette scholar, wrote the book's introduction. All of my D.C. friends owned the publication, which was filled with wonderfully textured colored photographs of musicians, festivals, dancers, and clubs.

Judith and Philip were zydeco fans, and had visited the black clubs before. Judith, who loved Beau Jocque, said she and her husband would be glad to accompany Diana and me to Richard's on Friday evening. I accepted her offer knowing their presence would make the experience more comfortable. I felt a bit ashamed, really, that I needed their company to cover my flank, as it were. But walking into Richard's with them at our side seemed like the right thing to do.

---

1. Philip Gould with Barry Jean Ancelet, *Cajun Music and Zydeco* (Baton Rouge: Louisiana State University Press, 1992).

We arrived at the club after ten, having cut through the prairie night on a highway that seemed to lead nowhere, until, on the left, a flashing road sign, like a rural lighthouse, pointed the way to Richard's. We probably would have found the club anyway, even without the sign, for the still evening air outside the place reverberated, as Beau Jocque's accordion sent thunder-claps of sound into the adjacent fields, beckoning people to come.

I walked into Richard's through a screened-door entrance, behind Philip, Judith, and Diana. The hall was packed, absolutely stuffed. Scores of couples filled the room, zydeco dancing in tight little slots as a house fan the size of a jet engine tried to cool the patrons. The dance floor was soft, made of wooden planks, and as dancers thumped its surface the ground pulsed up and down: the rhythmic shock waves of a zydeco earthquake.

Above it all, at the end of the room, stood Beau Jocque, all six-foot-six of him, a mountain of sweat and flesh and muscle. I had the impression he had to stoop in order to keep the top of his head from hitting a very low-slung ceiling. He sang in French and in English, and did so not so much with grace as with fortitude, delivering a deep, raspy voice with the charm of a bulldozer:

> *Ah, couche-couche!*
> *Give him cornbread,*
> *Give him cornbread,*

Give him cornbread,
Give him cornbread,
I want that cornbread!
Eh toi!

We were, as I had expected, the only white people in the room, and as we settled in we attracted our share of curious looks. But nobody was hostile. The mood was more or less indifferent.

I sat with Philip and Judith at a table for most of the evening, content to take in the dancers around me. Diana wandered off alone.

I was completely engaged by what I saw. I remember thinking how smooth the Creole dancers looked, and how controlled their movements were. Their style was mostly understated and contained, but their jumps and spins and open-position shines bespoke a certain elegance.

There was attitude, as well, a quiet pride, I thought, in what they were engaged in.

I especially liked the way some of the men constructed the closed position: the man's and woman's lead arms abandoned the normal outward extension at right angles to the body; instead, the man took the woman's right hand with his left, drew it across his torso, and planted it on his left hip, like a bolt. There it remained, beneath his palm, as his elbow jutted out backward in a splendid and defiant flash of masculinity.

As the night went on, I danced only once, with Judith. I wasn't prepared to approach a Creole woman yet with an offer to zydeco. This was a different dance culture, and I didn't know the rules. Not to mention the touchy issue of interracial dancing. As for Diana, she wasn't anywhere around, a point that Philip brought to my attention.

"Aren't you worried about your girlfriend?" he asked. The edge to his voice suggested that I should be, and the look in his eyes might just as well have said that white women shouldn't wander off alone in an establishment like this.

"Well, she's not my girlfriend," I replied. "I'm sure she can take care of herself."

I surveyed the club for Diana, and continued to do so for the next quarter hour. She wasn't anywhere around. She appeared at the end of the evening, apparently no worse for wear.

"Are you okay?" I asked. "Where have you been?"
"I'm fine."
She paused.
"I was outside talking with a friend."
We left it at that.

Diana and I became husband and wife the next evening. Our marriage had nothing to do with love. It was, instead, all about race. And anxiety of a different color.

We had agreed to visit Slim's Y-Ki-Ki that Saturday night, the zydeco dance club in Opelousas. Boozoo

Chavis would be onstage. And we would go to the place on our own, without the buffer that Judith and Philip had provided at Richard's Club.

Diana and I still really didn't know each other well. She had no knowledge of my history with panic disorder. And I had never told her about my apprehension regarding the black clubs. I'm not sure which form of anxiety would have been the more difficult to reveal. A psychiatric disorder is a hugely personal condition. Its revelation risks embarrassment and putting people off. I doubt Diana would have responded negatively had I told her, for she was an eminently kind woman. Her re-action probably would have mirrored Coco's: empathy, interest, support. But for the time being, I held on to my secret.

But shades of racism? This was an entirely differ-ent form of anxiety, one that crossed from the personal to public policy. My unease about visiting the black clubs was difficult enough to acknowledge to myself. Although it was right there, deep within, and it al-ways had been: a niggling voice in the pit of my belly that said, "Sorry, pal, whether you like it or not, black people scare you." Especially black men.

That's how I was raised: brought up in the insular eggshell of a white suburb in the sixties; conditioned by the culture around me to be afraid of a people I had met only in the local evening news, where Negroes—that was the moniker of the era—committed the crimes; frightened, perhaps even still, by the lingering, violent recollections of my youth, when nearby inner-city riots and shouts of "Black Power" made race war the current of newspaper pundits and a notion too real to ignore.

This was the prejudicial matter that had swayed much of white America, and had undeniably tainted my views. Now, having grown up, I certainly knew better. But still, it is difficult to disregard the past. Bias and stereotypes die awfully hard. So try as I might to shake them off, I carried them inside me when I entered Richard's Club, and as I prepared to make the trip to Slim's Y-Ki-Ki.

What I hadn't known was that Diana, too, was anxious about the issue of race. She had visited Slim's once before, on her previous Louisiana trip a few years back, and had gotten into trouble.

"I went with two white couples, and two of the guys were Cajuns," she said. "They told us not to dance with anybody else. They warned us not to dance with anybody else. But to me that was perplexing, because the black men there were phenomenal dancers, and I was there to have the opportunity to dance with someone local. I didn't want to pass that up.

"So I went ahead and danced with some Creole guys anyway. But one of the white men I was with kind of mixed it up with one of the guys I had danced with. And a black guy was kind of pestering me after I had danced with him. He wouldn't really leave me alone. And the guy I had come with was angry at me for dancing with the black guys. I was very confused about it all, because I hadn't realized that I would stand out so much in a place like that."

And what I didn't learn, until sometime later, was that Diana's troubles had continued on this trip, the night before, at Richard's Club.

"One of the guys I danced with at Richard's rubbed up against me with an erection," she said. "That made me feel really uncomfortable. I felt assaulted. He kept doing it. He wanted to pull me right up against his body, closer than you would normally dance zydeco. I just didn't want to dance that close to him. I didn't want to dance that close to anybody. I was finally able to get away from him. But whenever I went on the dance floor he kept trying to intercept me. It made it very difficult to dance with anybody else."

So Diana exited Richard's Club and spent much of the evening outside, which is why I never saw her.

In the car on the drive to Slim's Y-Ki-Ki, Diana asked if I would consent to be her husband for the evening. I agreed. If somebody pestered her, she could say she was with her spouse. She figured that a "married" white woman would be less likely to attract single black men.

We both were anxious, our antennas fully up, by the time we arrived at the club.

※

Slim's Y-Ki-Ki was an odd name for a South Louisiana prairie zydeco dance hall. The brick-wall front exterior looked nondescript and nothing like the beach in Honolulu. The establishment's signature road sign, however—which stood across the street from a Piggly Wiggly food store—did have a picture of a palm tree and a yellow setting sun. And inside there were more palm trees, painted on the walls in a madcap display of tropical artistry. The owner of the place, which had opened in 1947, clearly had a thing for things Hawaiian.

The centerpiece of Slim's was the music stage, which rose from the middle of a dusty wooden dance floor. When we walked in, Boozoo Chavis and the Majic Sounds had already started to play. Tables and dancers encircled the platform.

Again, Diana and I were the only white people there. Amazingly, our race seemed to work in our favor, as time and time again, as the evening progressed, people went out of their way to be friendly in order to make us feel at home.

"Hello, hello, come on in, glad to see y'all," said the lady at the door.

"Hey, where y'all from?" Boozoo shouted from the stage. By the end of the evening, Mr. Chavis had dedicated songs to Chicago and to Washington, D.C., a sign of pleasure on his part that we had traveled so far just to see him.

Diana and I danced a lot that night at Slim's Y-Ki-Ki, with each other (as husband and wife) and with local dancers, too. Buoyed and relieved by the kindness we had been shown, I managed to ask a few Creole women to dance, women who seemed to be there by themselves or with some lady friends. Not everyone said yes. One lady smiled but politely refused. Another just looked at me as if I were crazy. But two did agree to zydeco with me, and for that I was grateful. I can't say that the dances yielded any magic moments, but I was able to keep up.

My encounter with the local women did not pass unnoticed. After a round of dancing, one of the Creole patrons, a middle-aged black man wearing a cowboy hat, approached me from behind. He reached out and touched me on the shoulder. Since I was facing the other direction, his approach startled me, as did the grip he maintained near my neck. My heartbeat quickened, and a lifetime of racial stereotyping kicked in.

"Where is my wallet?" I wondered. "What is this guy going to do to me?"

I turned around and confronted my assailant, dreading some sort of confrontation.

He flashed me a wide grin and offered up a handshake. "You dance real good, you," he said, pumping my arm. "Where you from?"

I was stunned by what he had said, and ashamed by what I had been thinking.

"Washington, D.C.," I replied.

"Washington, D.C.? Well, how about that. Yeah, you dance real good."

As for Diana, she was never at a loss for partners that evening, as a bevy of Creole gentlemen callers of all ages, shapes, and sizes politely offered their hands for a dance. One elderly fellow, a septuagenarian nattily dressed in a jacket and tie, was particularly attracted to Diana. He was a smooth dancer, Diana said, and she didn't mind his attention.

"I finally had a good time dancing with black men," she said. "People were definitely interested in me, but in a much more respectful way than had been the case at Richard's Club. Before being asked to dance the men would sometimes point at you, making signs of a ring on their finger, asking if you were my husband. And I told people that you and I were married, and the evening went without incident. I finally got what I wanted. I was able to enjoy their dancing, and they were able to enjoy mine."

When the evening ended at two in the morning, Boozoo Chavis jumped off the stage and sauntered up to Diana and me. He gave each of us a bear hug, and thanked us again for coming.

Our spirits couldn't have been higher. We left Slim's and headed over to our car. A pea-soup fog filled the road, heightening the senses. Diana, who had driven, reached inside the pocket of her dress and fumbled for her keys. She pulled out a slip of paper instead, placed there surreptitiously by the feisty septuagenarian.

"My name is Joe," the note said. His telephone number followed. "Don't tell husband."

We laughed so hard that tears came to our eyes. And then we drove away.

The next morning, I went for a jog in Lafayette's Girard Park. The park would, with time, become one of my favorite places in Acadiana, excepting the Cajun and zydeco dance halls. Large oak trees provided ample shade and atmosphere. A stream snaked around the grounds. A nice running path encircled the terrain.

I had brought along a Walkman, earphones, still fresh memories of Boozoo Chavis, and a recording of Beau Jocque's latest album. As I eased into the run and my legs lost their morning stiffness, I noticed my pace picking up, keeping time, like a metronome, with the booming, repetitive riffs of Beau Jocque's accordion. I ran like that for fifty minutes, my stride literally merging with the music. As for my mind, it was completely at ease and as confident as it had ever been. It was a trancelike experience, really, a zydeco-fueled runner's high that announced, with an exclamation point, the fact that I had overcome panic disorder.

I thought about Diana during that run, and the great time we'd had the night before at Slim's; I thought about Coco Glass and Dr. Gilbert, my cotherapists, who had helped me to patch my life back together; but mostly I thought about zydeco music and dance, about the booming Beau Jocque tune that, stride after stride, was filling my brain and pulsing through my body. What I thought of next is pure cliché, and I hesitate to write it, but clichés are based in fact, and in fact, what I thought of next was this: Life doesn't get any better. Running on that carpet of zydeco, in the afterglow of Slim's Y-Ki-Ki, I felt strong, content, calm, happy. I finally felt completely cured.

I I

La Poussiere

Three weeks after Diana and I had left South Louisiana, a woman by the name of Zee Scott made the trip with a couple of her friends, Helene Greenwald and Matthew Bettenhausen. The group had been attending a conference in New Orleans and decided, once the meeting had ended, to travel to the Lafayette area to see the sights, to listen to some Cajun music, and, maybe, to dance. On a Saturday night, April 16, 1994, they headed over to Breaux Bridge and to La Poussiere, where Walter Mouton and his Cajun band were playing. They'd been told La Poussiere was a pleasant place to spend an evening.

When they arrived at the club, Helene left her companions in the car and went to the door to confirm the place was open. The group had tried to get in the night before, but the club was closed because of a private party. A La Poussiere employee told Helene that the club was indeed open to the public that evening, for a two-dollar cover charge. She returned to the car to get Zee, and the two women went back to the entrance while Matthew parked the vehicle.[1]

1. A fuller presentation of the La Poussiere case was broadcast on *Weekend All Things Considered* on August 20, 1995. The piece was written by Daniel Zwerdling and produced by me and Rebecca Davis.

"I went up to the door with Helene, and when we stood there the lady looked at us and she said, 'It's a private party,'" Zee recalled. "We walked away, and Helene, you know, was saying to herself , 'I don't really understand, she just told me it wasn't a private party.' And she said, 'You know, Zee, it's because you're black.' And I said, 'I know.'"

Helene and Matthew were white.

Helene decided to go back to the door to complain. En route, she saw three white women arriving at the club, and asked if they were there for a private party. They said they were not, and Helene saw them enter the facility after paying the two-dollar admission.

"And I'm standing there watching this," Helene said, "and the woman who had told me it was a private party looked at me, and I looked at her, and I basically said, 'This isn't a private party, is it?' And she said no. And I said, 'Well, why did you tell me and my friend it was a private party?' And she just looked at me. And I said, 'Is it because my friend is black?' And she said yes."

Zee was alarmed. "I was truly afraid," she said. "If she could look us in the face and tell us that you can't come in here because you're black, I mean, that meant she had the support of management and likely the support of the people that were going in there." And those were ingredients, Zee said, that could threaten violence.

Zee was also humiliated. "I mean, the color of my skin prevented my friends from having fun, from enjoying themselves. And that's embarrassing."

Zee Scott, whose formal first name is Zaldwaynaka, and her friends Helene Greenwald and Matthew Bettenhausen were assistant U.S. attorneys, based in Chicago. Zee was responsible for prosecuting criminal and civil rights cases. After returning home from Louisiana, the three lawyers decided to go after La Poussiere: they filed a complaint with the Civil Rights Division of the U.S. Department of Justice.

The Federal Bureau of Investigation began an inquiry. One white couple and one black couple, all FBI undercover agents, subsequently were dispatched to La Poussiere on a Saturday night. The white couple entered the club after paying a cover charge. Thirty minutes later, on the same evening, the African American undercover agents were refused entry, again on the grounds that a private party was being held.

Zee Scott, Helene Greenwald, and Matthew Bettenhausen sued La Poussiere for violating the Civil Rights Act of 1964. The Justice Department filed a separate civil action, accusing La Poussiere of following a pattern, practice, and policy of refusing admission to African American citizens. Deval Patrick, then assistant attorney general for civil rights, said: "Over three decades ago, Congress spoke for all decent Americans by making it illegal to exclude people from places like this because of their skin color. It is startling that thirty years later this club still hasn't gotten the message."

In court papers, La Poussiere initially denied the allegations of discrimination. On the eve of the trial, however, in February 1996, the case was settled: La Poussiere admitted it had been unlawfully turning away blacks and pledged to end its discriminatory policies. The club owners paid Zee Scott and her friends an undisclosed amount of money in damages. The owners agreed to undergo training on civil rights issues. And they posted a sign outside the nightclub's door. It read:

> Welcome to La Poussiere. Open to all members of the public regardless of race or color. If you feel you have been discriminated against, let us know and write or call collect: Housing and Civil Enforcement Section, Civil Rights Division, U.S. Dept. of Justice, P.O. Box 65998, Washington, D.C. 20035–5998. (202) 514–4713.

Sometime after the lawsuits had been settled, somebody pasted a small billboard on the sign, right next to the Justice Department's address. It was an advertisement for "Bayou"-brand boudin and cracklin, local delicacies made, respectively, of rice and pork sausage and of fried strips of pork skin. Interestingly, both whites and blacks like to eat these foods.

The La Poussiere litigation was first and foremost about racism and discrimination, which endure, as the facts showed, in not so subtle ways, even in public accommodations. But the case also revealed something about the nature of social dance, something that I observed as I returned to South Louisiana again and again in the years after my first visit with Diana.

Dancing, regardless of the venue, can stir up men

and women. As innocent, as anxiety reducing, as fun as social dance may be, what you have, at bottom line, is the potentially inflammatory act of males and females touching one another. This, in turn, can fuel the emotions and spark some baser human impulses, such as jealousy and lust, mistrust and suspicion. These feelings can and do exist in a homogenous environment, in which everyone on the dance floor belongs to the same race. When the races mingle, things can get more complex.

That complexity was the backdrop to Zee Scott's reception at La Poussiere. That complexity, and the need to understand it, would dominate my visits to South Louisiana for nearly two years. The anxiety that had impaired my mental health was gone. But I realized, as I returned to the black zydeco dance halls, that the anxiety I had experienced about issues of race remained, my good time with Diana at Slim's Y-Ki-Ki notwithstanding. And it propelled me into a journalistic examination of interracial dancing in South Louisiana.

La Poussiere, as it turned out, did not always refuse entry to African Americans. Had Zee Scott gone there on a Wednesday evening, she probably would have been admitted. Wednesday nights were bingo nights at La Poussiere, and blacks had shared bingo tables there with whites for years. But on Saturday nights, when the dancing started, that was another matter. The distinction, which I didn't immediately understand, was explained to me by two longtime Lafayette-area residents, Donald Fusilier and his wife, Marella.

The Fusiliers were a handsome, articulate African American couple on the early edge of middle age. They lived with their eleven-year-old daughter in a well-to-do house in a racially mixed neighborhood in Carencro, just outside Lafayette. They described Acadiana as a quiet and peaceful part of the country. A lovely place to live.

Donald was something of a Creole-community local hero: he was chief prosecutor for the city of Lafayette, the first African American to hold that position. He served in the post at the time of the La Poussiere litigation, although he did not work on the case. But a lifetime in Lafayette—he grew up there—and three years at the center of the city's justice system put Donald Fusilier in a position to know about the region's attitudes and practices regarding race.

Donald said he was not surprised by Zee Scott's treatment at La Poussiere. The media, he said, portray Acadiana as a place filled with friendly Cajuns and Creoles. "And there are a lot of friendly people, and there are friendly Cajuns, so to speak. But if you go a little deeper you're going to find a lot of hatred and a lot of racism. We have to live with it day in and day out. It doesn't stop. It's so common. It's so normal in this area that it's funny."

Donald said local Creoles understand one enduring, simple fact of life: there are some white establishments in Acadiana that do not want their business. La Poussiere, he said, was among them. "The way we react to it is we don't go to the club," he said. "Had this black lady who worked for the Justice Department called me and talked to me, I would have told her, 'Hey, you're wasting your time. You're either going to get beat up or thrown out of the club.' It just happens, okay? It happens all the time."

But what about bingo? I asked. Black people go to La Poussiere on Wednesday nights to play bingo, and they mingle there with whites.

"In bingo you're not socializing," Donald said. "You're not trying to talk to the white girl, or you're not trying to talk to the black girl or the black man. There's no interracial dating, okay? You don't even talk to each other. You play bingo and you try to win your money and you take your money and go home."

But dancing, especially at an establishment like La Poussiere, that was something different. "That's dangerous," Marella explained, "because there's socializing. You know, 'Are you going to take my girlfriend from me? You, black guy, are you going to take my white girlfriend from me?' That is what they are looking at and what they're seeing at that particular moment in time, on that dance floor, in that club. That's what they're thinking."

In short, black men and women could not dance at La Poussiere because Cajun regulars feared that black patrons might steal their white partners away. That was the opinion of the Fusiliers.

It was a point of view that Barry Jean Ancelet, the University of Louisiana at Lafayette folklorist, would not dispute. "Socialization has traditionally been closed, especially by whites, and especially in situations where courtship is likely," he said. And courtship, he said, is likely on the dance floor.

The dance hall "has long functioned as a primary setting for courtship within traditional Louisiana French society," Ancelet explained. It "remains as closed as the universities, lunch counters, and polling booths once were."

Ancelet spoke about interracial dancing in South Louisiana in a presentation to the American Folklore Society in 1996.

Ancelet pointed out that dance-hall discrimination has sometimes been color blind. It has even been found among Cajuns themselves. "Traditional Cajun society has historically been extremely territorial, and dance halls have long been one of the most important definers of local community," he said. "Where people went to dance on Saturday nights identified their neighborhood or regional allegiance as much as and maybe even more than where they went to school or to church. Terrible fights over someone from another village dancing with the local girls was not uncommon. These sorts of conflicts have diminished, though not disappeared, over the years."

But for Cajuns, Ancelet said, interracial dancing has always touched a different, more sensitive nerve. There was and remains a clear "boundary between the races in matters of courtship and kinship." Blacks and whites simply did and mostly do not dance together. To do so risked romance, which in turn could lead to a mixing of the races.

In far less tolerant times, breaching the sanction on interracial dancing, even an innocent breach, could produce terrible consequences. Ancelet recalled the story of a Creole accordionist named Amédé Ardoin. Ardoin is considered a pioneer of both Cajun and Creole music, an artist whose meshing of French and African melodies and rhythms laid the groundwork for the contemporary Cajun and zydeco sound. During the 1920s and 1930s, Ardoin performed with a Cajun fiddler named Dennis McGee. Their interracial partnership was tolerated despite the constraints of Jim Crow segregation. Ardoin was popular everywhere, and the two men were allowed to perform at Cajun dances—where all the dancers were white.

Ancelet said Ardoin "eventually died as a result of the brutal beating he received at the hands of a few indignant white men after he accepted a handkerchief from a white girl to wipe the sweat from his brow during a Saturday-night dance. It mattered not that she was the daughter of his white employer who knew him as a friend of the family, and that she had simply reacted instinctively in a humane way to relieve his distress from the heat, as she would have had they been out in the fields picking cotton. But they weren't in the fields picking cotton. They were in a dance hall where dancing and courtship were at stake. And the friendship ties he enjoyed with the host family did not protect him from the wrath of the protectors of white purity."

Ancelet concluded that even now, "the old-time Cajun music dance hall has remained a bastion of segregation" in South Louisiana. In significant part that is because of white attitudes, which can still be unwelcoming toward blacks. But even in some of the larger, more urban Cajun clubs where blacks might be greeted warmly at the door, there is little reason to think that African American dancers would want to show up anyway.

"With rare exception, Creoles have shown little interest in attending such places," Ancelet said, echoing the views of Donald and Marella Fusilier: People do not go where they think they are not wanted. People tend to stay with their own. In South Louisiana, that means that Cajuns go to Cajun dances, and Creoles go to zydeco. When the exception does surface, however, when a Creole shows up at a Cajun event, racism can still taint the results, even in the aftermath of the La Poussiere litigation.

As in the case of Geno Delafose, the zydeco recording artist.

Geno was a young musician in his early twenties

when I first met him in Washington, D.C. His father, John Delafose, had been a major force in zydeco music until his death in 1994. Geno, who had played drums in his father's band, had also become an accomplished accordionist. He formed his own ensemble, the French Rockin' Boogie, even before his dad passed away. Geno and his band played frequently in the Washington area, at the Glen Echo Spanish Ballroom, and at Tornado Alley. He got to know many of the regular dancers, including me. "Whenever you're in Louisiana, come on by and visit at the ranch," he said. Like Diana before me, I took him up on the offer.

Geno was born and still lives in the cradle of the South Louisiana prairie, in a small rural town called Eunice, about an hour's drive west of Lafayette. His ranch, called the Double-D (named for Delafose the father, then Delafose the son) is seven acres of flatland tucked well off the main road. "Cross the tracks, go past the bayou, and turn left onto the gravel road just past the church." That's how you get there, according to Geno Delafose.

Directions notwithstanding, the place was difficult to find. When I pulled up to what I thought was the proper location, I asked a farmhand if Geno Delafose was around, just to be sure I had found the Double-D.

"He's right over there, by the cows," the man replied.

Geno was standing near the cattle pen, looking more like a snatch of prairie tumbleweed than a zydeco music sensation. He was hunched over, trying to hitch an empty trailer to a truck. He wore a dusty pair of jeans, a sleeveless blue T-shirt, and a baseball cap that said "Rodeo is Life." An impatient cow mooed angrily nearby. "He hasn't been fed yet," Geno said.

The Double-D was a working ranch, equipped with twenty-six head of cattle, four horses, one dog, and a faded blue Ford tractor. "It's not a very big moneymaking thing," Geno said, "but it's a great pastime, and I love it."

Geno has a kind, handsome face—a soft, accessible face—with easygoing eyes and a boyish grin. He lives in the house he grew up in, a modest, one-level white wood-frame structure surrounded by pastures, fields of soybean and rice, and a white picket fence. We sat down to talk at a table in his large, cluttered kitchen, filled with the hodgepodge of everyday life—cereal boxes, rice cooker, coffeemaker, heaps of mail—along with the stuff that attached to Geno Delafose: a couple of cowboy hats hanging on pegs on the cabinet doors, one white and one black; a handful of accordions strewn across the linoleum floor; a rack of jacketless old 45s that belonged to his father, their black vinyl surfaces scarred from ancient encounters with turntable needles; and a belly-high stack of compact discs—zydeco and Cajun music, by various artists.

It was Cajun music, and Geno's affection for it, that made him distinct among zydeco bandleaders. He often performed tunes that were more apt to suggest a Cajun jig or two-step than the close-in zydeco dance.

"There's a lot of Cajun music in my music," he acknowledged.

I asked him if he goes to the Cajun dance clubs.

"Well, there is a racial issue, and I must admit, there are a lot of times I want to go and hear some bands play, and I may even go to the club and then get there and, you know, it just doesn't feel right. I love the music. I play the music. And you know, anywhere outside the state of Louisiana I don't have a problem going to hear a Cajun band. But you know, here, sometimes it's kind of hard. And I don't want no trouble, because it's so easy to get in trouble and it's so hard to get out of."

Geno found some trouble on a Saturday night in January 1998, when two of his white friends, Christine Balfa and her husband, Dirk Powell, performed with their band, Balfa Toujours, at Da Office, a small Cajun dance club in Basile, Louisiana, ten minutes up the road from the Delafose ranch.

Christine is another of Dewey Balfa's daughters.

"And they asked me to come by and hear them play," Geno said. "So I was not thinking anything of it. I went, me and my mom, and when I walked in the door, I didn't know if there was a cover charge or not. There was nobody collecting. So I just walked in, and some guy came up to me and asked me, 'How are you doing?'"

According to Dirk Powell, the man who approached Geno was not the club's owner, but one of its patrons.

"I told him, fine," Geno said. "And he said, 'You know, I think you ought to leave, because we don't mix here too much. You know, if you don't want no trouble you should go.'"

Dirk Powell said the man then tried to pressure the club's owner to force Geno off the premises.

"And that was shocking to me," Geno said, because he had thought times had changed. Eleven years earlier, when he was sixteen years old, Geno had gone with some friends to a Cajun music hall in Eunice called the Liberty Theater. "We went and listened to some band play," he recalled, "and after the show a guy came out plain and asked me, 'Were you dancing there with those white ladies?' And I said yeah. He said, 'Well, you know, you need to stick with your own kind.' And that really just shocked the hell out of me, and it pissed me off a lot, too. But I just walked away from it. And I thought that stuff was just about over with. And then here, here I am, twenty-seven years old, and the same thing happens again."

Geno said the Basile incident had a happy ending, however. When Christine found out what Geno had encountered, she invited him to come up onstage and play. "And I played about forty-five minutes, and people just went crazy in that club. They were dancing and everything, and just stood around the stage, and you know, it was a wonderful feeling."

The next Monday, which was Martin Luther King Jr. Day, Christine Balfa received a call from the management of another nearby Cajun club, the Main Street

Lounge. Balfa Toujours had been scheduled to play there later in the week. According to Christine Balfa, the management was calling because word had gotten out that Balfa Toujours had invited Geno Delafose on-stage at Da Office.

"They said, 'We've heard rumors. Are you going to have any blacks in the band when you play here?' I replied, 'If any of my friends come, I'm sure not going to tell them they aren't welcome, no matter what color they are.' The Main Street then replied, 'Well, we are going to have to cancel, then. People in Basile are just like that, and it will never change.'"

Balfa Toujours was fired from their gig. And according to Dirk Powell, there are still Cajuns in and around Basile who will not attend a Balfa Toujours dance because of what happened at Da Office, and because of Christine's friendship with Geno Delafose.

(When I called the Main Street Lounge—well after the incident took place—to get their side of the story, a woman who identified herself as the manager said she didn't know anything about Christine Balfa and Geno Delafose. "I don't have French music here since I took over," she said. She hung up on me as I was trying to determine whether she had been running the club in January 1998.)

If Creoles generally have shown little interest in attending Cajun dances, Cajuns have been equally uninterested in flocking to zydeco events. Again, a legacy of segregation and a predisposition to partake in one's own culture have been high walls to overcome. But there are some in the Cajun community who have crossed the color line, and their reception at the black clubs has been, for the most part, positive.

Folklorist Barry Ancelet, who grew up in Lafayette, recalled that during the 1970s — "troubled times" racially in South Louisiana — he and a few of his white friends used to go hear Clifton Chenier at the Blue Angel, one of the black dance venues.

"There was ongoing tension in the community over the lessons of coming together at the water fountains, on the buses, and at the lunch counters," Ancelet said. "Yet the prevailing sentiment in the club was repeated by almost everyone: 'Don't worry about anything, baby. Everybody's welcome here. You won't have no trouble.' I realized later that we were perfectly safe there because unlike Cajun dance-hall patrons, those Creole patrons were not interested in enforcing barriers. They seemed delighted instead that barriers may be coming down. It is also undeniable that it would have been disastrous for something to happen to us in that club. The wrath of the white community would have fallen on the patrons and the owners as it had on Clifton's predecessor, Amédé Ardoin."

More than thirty years later, as the popularity and reach of zydeco music expand, whites continue to be welcomed at the black zydeco clubs, and in increasing numbers. Some of these patrons are open-minded Cajuns who simply love the music. In Lafayette there is even a zydeco dance class taught by white instructors.

Most of the dancers, however, are out-of-towners, people like me, who discovered zydeco in the diaspora and were drawn to South Louisiana to experience the music in its original setting.

One of the most popular places to do so is the annual Southwest Louisiana Zydeco Music Festival, which takes place each Labor Day weekend on a dusty field qua dance floor in a place called Plaisance, north of Lafayette. "Ninety percent of the whites you see dancing are not from the state of Louisiana," said Paul Scott, one of the festival's organizers. And the remaining 10 percent, he said, are from elsewhere in the state—primarily New Orleans—and not from the local Cajun community.

The festival was conceived as a vehicle for local Creoles to celebrate their culture, and according to Paul Scott there has been, at least among a few Creoles, a backlash of sorts against the incursion of white dancers at the festival and onto the dance floors of local zydeco clubs. There is a belief, he said, that whites may be hijacking Creole culture, and profiting from it.

To illustrate the point, Paul told me the story of a friend of his, an African American, who came to him one day in an agitated mood, waving a local newspaper. The zydeco festival had just occurred, and there was a photograph on the paper's front page of some of the dancers who had attended.

"And he said to me, 'What's wrong with that picture?'" Paul recalled. "And I said, 'Is it the dust, or a little accident we had out there?' And he said, 'No. There ain't no black people in this picture. I thought this was a black festival.'"

I came upon a similar sentiment once when I visited KRVS-FM, "Radio Acadie," the NPR member station in Lafayette. I went there to interview John Broussard, who was the Creole host of a popular Saturday-morning zydeco show. The show was broadcast mainly in French. I wanted to speak with Broussard about zydeco dancing and its role in the Creole community. Broussard initially agreed to the interview, but when I showed up, he said he would not proceed. He voiced concern about outsiders exploiting his culture for profit.

Paul Scott attributed these attitudes to a lingering resentment by some in the Creole community to past instances of white people exploiting black culture. He recalled the story of Big Mama Thornton, a black blues singer from Alabama who had recorded the song "Hound Dog"—as in "You ain't nothin' but a hound dog"—only to have had it popularized, at great personal profit, by a white singer named Elvis Presley.

"History is like nature; it has seasons and it repeats itself," Paul said. "You want to be protected because in the past you've gotten things, not so much taken away, but mainstreamed, or reinvented. I think a lot of blacks have that fear. They think: 'Hey, look, this is ours.'"

Paul said these concerns were not shared by the black zydeco club owners, however, or by the zydeco bands, who in fact benefit financially from white outsiders coming to Louisiana to dance. "The venues are black owned. And the bands getting paid are black. I think club owners realize that if this white person comes in here, one, he's going to spend money; two, he wants to be here; three, he ain't going to cause no trouble; and four, he's going to bring more people. So it's an economic thing, and we're going to make sure you have a good time."

There was, at least initially, resistance among some black patrons to the appearance of white dancers in the zydeco clubs. Roy Carrier, the zydeco musician, owns a small rural dance hall called the Offshore Lounge in Lawtell, Louisiana.

"Whites started coming to my club in the late 1980s," he said. "People would tell me, 'What are you letting these white trash in here for?' There was a lot of black prejudice with some of the regulars at my club back then. And I would tell them, 'I don't care about white and I don't care about black. All I care about is green. I want to make money, so get lost.'"

The Offshore Lounge, to my mind, was the most interesting zydeco dance club in South Louisiana. It was, for one, the most difficult to find, situated, like an afterthought, thirty yards north of the Southern Pacific train tracks a few blocks west of "Matt's Museum— Best in State" on U.S. 190 in Lawtell. It was known for its Thursday-night jams, wherein Roy Carrier, a veteran accordionist, would tutor younger musicians in the art of zydeco. It was also the place in which I learned that a white guy like me can sometimes have trouble finding a Creole woman dance partner under the age of sixty.

The club was the embodiment of ramshackle. It stood, barely, like a tumbledown shanty on a patch of flatland, propped precariously in the vertical position by some hardy pillars and the grace of God. The interior space was rectangular, filled in the middle by a large wooden dance floor. At one end was the stage, a stumpy platform framed by some garden trellis, which hung from the ceiling and rose from the floor. The latticework was tattered, as if by shrapnel. The stage was backed by a sheaf of wrinkled aluminum foil, strung out like wallpaper, makeshift designed, I assumed, to reflect the music of Roy Carrier and the Night Rockers out into the hall.

On the evening I was there, the dance floor was half-filled with Creole couples. At center court was Zydeco Joe, a rail-thin senior dressed in a tie, red jacket, and faded yellow pants, cavorting around like a jumping bean. Two dozen people sat in plastic chairs at the Formica-topped tables that lined the dance-floor perimeter. A pool table stood in the far corner of the club, a courteous sop to the nondancer. A bar was attached to the opposite wall. Attached to the bar was a handful of Creole men, dressed in sleeveless T-shirts and baseball caps, sipping beers and chatting. The chirping sound of crickets punctuated their conversation. The insects inhabited the club along with the patrons.

I went to the Offshore Lounge club with Jane Jeffries, a onetime Washingtonian who, at the time, was living in Baton Rouge. Jane was a political consultant, and she had come south to work on a Louisiana gubernatorial campaign. She was also a zydeco fanatic and had logged more hours in the Creole clubs than any white woman I knew.

Jane had a great time that evening. Creole men of all ages approached her with invitations to dance, and, on occasion, with propositions for something more.

"They always give you the same three questions," Jane said. "'Are you married? Did you come here with someone? Do you want to sleep with me?' I danced with one very old gentleman, he must have been over seventy, and he said at the end of our dance—and these were the only words he spoke—'You know, I live alone.'"

None of this bothered Jane, who always handled the propositions with humor and great aplomb, politely explaining to her suitors that, no, thank you very much, she didn't want to sleep with them, but she appreciated the offer and did enjoy the dance.

I later surveyed my other Washington women friends who had danced at the Creole clubs in South Louisiana and found that they, like Jane, were never at a loss for Creole partners, and that they, too, had fielded the three questions on more than one occasion.

Some of these women believed—as Diana Steele had before them—that they were pursued solely because of their race. Jane, for instance, was told by one of her Creole friends that "some black guys here in South Louisiana think if a white lady talks to them, the lady wants to sleep with them." Another Washington woman said she was seen as a racial trophy, her dance-floor popularity the product of "one-upmanship, especially among the younger Creole guys."

"A lot of times these guys have a night out with the boys, and it's a bit of a competitive sport to see who you can dance with," she said. "White women are particularly a target. It's prestigious to dance with a white woman because only now, with the barriers of segregation changing, is that seen as possible."

Other Washington women dancers said gender, not race, is what made them stand out. "There probably are some Creole men who are especially eager to dance with white women because they are 'from out of town,'" my friend Linda acknowledged. "But I think any woman is popular on the dance floors of South Louisiana. Women are popular in bars, period. It is assumed that they are single and there to meet men. The local women are always asked to dance, but some of them refuse to dance with certain men because they know them and don't like them, or don't like the way they dance, or because the men are married. But we out-of-towners don't have any history. Many of us are not married, and we're there looking to dance with anyone and everyone. So I don't believe the popularity of out-of-towners is due to race."

Paul Scott, the zydeco-festival organizer, agreed. He rolled his eyes and laughed when I asked him whether Creole men reserved the "three questions" for white women only. It is not a question of race, he said. It is a matter of gender, of romantic possibility, the old give-and-take of the birds and the bees.

"It's a social dance and the guys are being social," he explained.

"Social?" I said. "You mean to say that the same guys who ask those three questions to white women—"

"Will ask them to anybody," he said.

"They'll ask the three questions to black women, too?"

"Yes indeed, yes indeed. Oh yes, indeed."

"Because that's the way they socialize?"

"Yeah, yeah. It's a club. It's a way of meeting people. It's a social event."

"So in your view this behavior, the three questions, is not targeted to white women dancers. It's just targeted to women, period?"

"Period. Period."

While Jane was dancing nonstop to the locomotion of Roy Carrier's zydeco accordion that evening, I was mostly stewing in the corner, having failed, with one exception, to find myself a Creole partner. It was not, to be sure, for the lack of effort. I asked a dozen local women to join me on the dance floor. My only affirmative respondent was a lonely gray-haired senior in a floral-print dress. I'm certain the Offshore Lounge had never seen a more curious-looking couple: me, a forty-two-year-old bearded Jew, leading a dainty but frail old lady of African lineage through the slow-pause-quick-quicks of the zydeco dance.

At the evening's end, Jane was exultant and I was upset. We had been the only white faces in the club, yet our experiences had been totally different. She had been embraced on the dance floor, and I had been shut out. The reason, I figured, had little to do with my dancing skills. It was, I thought, about race. As it turned out, I was right. And I was wrong.

"The reason why they won't dance with someone like you is because of the simple fact: there's a saying 'white people can't dance,'" said Dwight Carrier, Roy's nephew.

Dwight Carrier stood outside the Offshore Lounge, nursed a Budweiser, and tried to make sense of my dance-floor conundrum. Dwight, twenty-four, was a zydeco accordionist in his own right. He grew up in one of South Louisiana's preeminent Creole music families, and had danced since he was ten, when his mother taught him how to zydeco.

"You're telling me that black people down here assume that white guys don't know how to dance simply because they're white?" I asked.

"They have no rhythm," Dwight said matter-of-factly. "They have no soul. You see, in order to dance to zydeco music you have to have the feeling. You have to feel the music. You feel it from the heart.

"I grew up with it," Dwight declared, lifting an eyebrow that pointedly said, "and you did not." "So it comes from the heart every time I dance."

As I got to know other Creole dancers, Dwight's explanation grew less surprising. I heard it over and over again. At Thibodeaux's, a Lake Charles hall, a Creole woman invited me to dance only after she had seen me zydeco with a Washington friend. "You dance like a black person!" she exclaimed. "I was so amazed. White guys usually don't dance like us. But you were great."

Another Creole acquaintance similarly told me: "For a white man, boy, you sure can zydeco."

Keisha Robertson, a twenty-one-year-old Eunice resident, conveyed the same message. "You have trouble finding Creole partners because people stereotype," she said. "And black people stereotype white people as not knowing how to dance."

So Creole women did not want to dance with me because I was white, per se. They rejected me because they had come to the dance hall to dance, and figured, based on their experience in life, that I didn't know what I was doing. Why waste time with an inept dancer?

The same rationale guided thinking at the clubs back home, at Tornado Alley and Glen Echo Park, where most of the patrons were white. Few of my friends there were ever especially eager to dance with a partner who couldn't hold their own. Unless the partner was attractive, and "socializing" became the driving force. Then we'd make exceptions—some of us, at least—in the name of seeking romance. I had been guilty of that transgression any number of times, targeting good-looking women on the dance floors of Washington, D.C.

What I ultimately realized—though I suppose it should have been obvious—is that Creole men and Creole women probably behaved pretty much like me. They were driven, I suspected, by the same motivations, by the same desire to dance with a skilled partner, by the same desire to make the acquaintance of a handsome partner and to enjoy his or her companionship on the dance floor. As for Diana Steele, Jane Jeffries, and my other Washington women friends, who happened to be white, they met all of the criteria: they were skilled dancers, nice looking, pleasant to be with. And that is why, when they zydeco danced in the Louisiana clubs, the Creole men found them so appealing. No wonder. So did I.

On my last trip to South Louisiana, I sat down with a handful of Creole dancers to talk about zydeco. We met in Opelousas, at the offices of the zydeco festival. I wanted to hear firsthand about Creole rules of dance-floor etiquette: what kind of behavior they expected on their dance floor from other dancers within their community.

James Douglas, forty-seven, was a construction worker who lived in Lawtell. "To me it's respect the next dancer," he said. "That's my number-one rule. If you do bump them accidentally, say, 'I'm sorry, excuse me.' Or after the dance apologize."

What about asking a woman to dance?

"To me," James said, "if a man comes into a club—whether he's married or not—if he sees a young lady he should say: 'Excuse me, before I ask you for this dance, I'd like to know whether you're married or with someone tonight. Is it okay that we dance?' Or a very respectable way to ask a married woman to dance is to go up to her husband and ask his permission."

"But you have those who go to the extreme," James said. "If the lady refuses, some of these guys will continue to nag, even though they've been told no. They continue until you have enough of it. Then you have to put your foot down."

Carolyn Douglas, James's wife, agreed. Carolyn, forty-two, was a grocery-store worker. "There are some men that come up to your table and want to grab and pull you onto the floor. I don't go for that at all. You tell them no, and they still come back and say, 'Come on, come on.' I mean, no means no, you know?"

Keisha Robertson, the Eunice dancer, was attractive and single and accustomed to going to the Creole clubs alone. I asked her if she had been targeted by overly aggressive dancers. "Some guys want to get a little bit too close for comfort," she said. "It does happen, and I say, 'Can you just back up because I'm uncomfortable.' I tell them that. Not in a mean way. I just let them know how I'm feeling, and they have to respect that. They normally back up. But if they come and grab and all—uh-uh, none of that. I didn't come here for that. I'm not a rag doll."

I had expected I might hear something unfamiliar, some distinctly African American point of view from these Creole dancers. Instead, what I heard was common sense and the golden rule.

After the discussion had ended, I dropped by the office of Paul Scott, the zydeco-festival organizer. Paul was a big man, both in size and in generosity of spirit. He was also the most open, thoughtful, and articulate person I had met in South Louisiana's black community. He had a way of focusing my thoughts.

"When a white person like myself comes to South Louisiana to zydeco," I said, "you think about many things. You think primarily about this wonderful music and this wonderful dance form. I mean, that's why you've come here. But the racial thing is obvious. Particularly at the beginning, when you're anxious, when you're getting your dance legs, so to speak, and finding your bearings on a zydeco dance floor in a black club. There's a learning curve. And I can tell you that white dancers think about it and worry about it, about how they will be treated, about how to behave properly, about the local rules of dance-floor etiquette."

"That fear you have, you brought it with you," Paul said. "At the zydeco clubs, black, white, it don't make a difference. You walk into the club with the fear. But the whole time you're down there, it's a positive experience because nothing negative happens. So when you leave you say, 'Well, you know, I was worried for nothing.'"

"So how do you react," I said, "when white guys like me tell you they're a little nervous about going into the black zydeco clubs?"

"They'll get over it. They'll get over it," he said. "Because they'd never come back here if they didn't."

12
Wildman

Of all the zydeco dancers I had ever seen in South Louisiana, nobody filled up the dance floor like Wildman Joe Potier:

JAMES DOUGLAS: He does aerobic zydeco.

CAROLYN DOUGLAS: No. Chiropractic zydeco.

KEISHA ROBERTSON: His name pretty much says it all. Wildman.

ME: Have you ever danced with him?

KEISHA: Yes.

ME: What's that like?

KEISHA: Wild. It is wild. I was like, okay, what is he gonna do next? I like to think of myself as a pretty good dancer, but when I got on the floor with him I was like, "okay, okay, okay." And I looked at what was going on, and my legs were in the air and my head was down on the ground.

CAROLYN: The first time I seen him dance I seen him on the floor, and I said, "What's he doin'? What's he doin'?" He dives on the floor. He jumps back up. You just had to look.

JAMES: From one second to another I don't think he knows what he's doing. It just goes with him. It's in him. The music just takes over in him.

CAROLYN: Energy. Energy. A lot of energy.

JAMES: Pure, raw energy.

Psychiatrists can offer up a handful of remedies for panic disorder. There are pills of various shapes and colors, antianxiety drugs that calm the brain. There is talk therapy, my course of treatment, which opens up the patient's mind to alternative ways of thinking, behaving, and processing emotions. And there are combinations of these two approaches. I suspect, however, that for psychiatrists in South Louisiana there is a third prescription: Go out and get to know the Wildman, because when you are with him on the dance floor, panic panics, anxiety withers, and what you're left with is nothing but wide eyes, good feelings, and zydeco-laced smiles.

I first spoke with Cealton Joseph Potier before I saw him dance. And for those who had only chatted with the man and had never watched him zydeco—if such people existed, I couldn't say for sure—Joe Potier, a.k.a. the Wildman, probably would have ranked among the gentlest souls in Acadiana.

"I work with mentally retarded kids for a living," he told me as we settled into a conversation at my Lafayette motel room one evening. "I work with the elderly, too. And I'm a professional mechanic. And a professional dancer."

Joe Potier, as he's known off the dance floor, has the soft-spoken manner of a church Sunday reverend and the clean-shaven face of an angel. His eyes are endearing and his smile genuine and sweet. He showed up neatly dressed in the tamest of apparel: a baseball cap, bright-red shirt, black slacks, and polished leather shoes. He looked like a scholarly thirty-year-old graduate student, although he was actually forty-five. I liked him instantly. Joe was an honest-to-goodness really nice guy.

"I'm from a little place called Parks, Louisiana," he said. "That's where I first saw zydeco."

Parks is a small Creole farming town on Bayou Teche, southeast of Lafayette. Wildman said his uncle had owned Dauphine's, a famous dance club there. It was the young Joe Potier's childhood playground.

"It was one of the first clubs that Clifton Chenier would play zydeco at. My grandmother lived next door to the place. So did my aunt. Me and my cousins, we liked the music but we was too young to go in, so we used to stand on barrels and watch the old people dance through the screen and window. Then we would go and do the same thing outside, behind the club. We would kill the grass all over. The next day the grass was dead."

Joe Potier smiled at the childhood recollection, remembering, perhaps for the first time in a long time, the genealogy of his connection to zydeco dance. Joe had always been a gifted dancer, a kid whose arms and legs moved naturally to music, just as surely as his lungs drew in air. When he was a six-year-old child, his father put him to work.

"I'm from a family of twelve, and it was pretty hard times," he said. "When I'd get home from school my dad would say, 'Son, come on over here. I want you to dance for my friends.' So I used to dance, and they used to throw me nickels and quarters and stuff, and that paid for my lunch and my milk or extra cookies."

By the time he had entered high school, Joe Potier had given up on zydeco. *Soul Train* was on the air, and other dance forms were more popular among his peers. Like rock and roll and disco. It was disco that gave Joe Potier his sobriquet. "People just saw me on the dance floor, and they called me wild. I have never called myself that, though."

Joe continued to dance in college, at Southern University in Baton Rouge, and it was there that his celebrity grew. He performed in a rock-and-roll dance troupe that competed on the college circuit: at Texas Southern, Mississippi Valley, and Jackson State. He also became a disco regular on a locally televised dance show, on channel 33.

With time, Joe Potier tired of the local disco scene. The clubs had become too rough, he said, too unpleasant, too often the venue for car thieves and drug dealers and lowlifes.

"So I went to a dance in the country one day," he recalled. It was a zydeco trail ride, a uniquely Creole institution wherein family and friends gather on horseback and trot across the prairie, stopping here and there for refreshments, and ultimately for social dance.

"And they had this guy who was a great zydeco dancer," Joe said. "He was inspiring. Everybody enjoyed watching him. He was the center of attention. Like, he had lines of ladies to dance with all the time. And I said, you know what, I'm going to be that guy one day."

On an Easter Sunday afternoon, at the Big Hat Club north of Lafayette, Joe Potier, then thirty-six, returned to the zydeco dance floor. "Everybody was laughing at me," he said. "They had seen me on TV and said, 'Man, you're a disco dancer, you're not no zydeco dancer. How in the world are you going to come in and zydeco?' They didn't know my past history, and I said, 'Y'all don't worry about it. Today's the day I'm going to get back into zydeco.'"

Joe Potier became a zydeco sensation, a one-man dance-floor event. He often appeared on *Zydeco Extravaganza,* the half-hour televised dance show, set in the local Creole clubs. The program initially aired at noon on Sundays. It was hugely popular, so much so that its viewers stayed away from church in order not to miss it. "So they put it on Saturday mornings at 11:30, right before *Soul Train,*" Joe said.

Joe Potier developed an eclectic dancing style that blended traditional Creole steps with disco, hip-hop, and rock and roll. He called it his "zydeco jambalaya." "You go in there, you try to do a few basics, and you add your own. The most important thing is to have fun."

Wildman's signature move took place on the ground. It was anxiety antithesis. "The part when I dance on my knees," he explained. "I dance on my knees. And I dance on my back. People, they call that wild."

In 1992, Joe Potier made it to the movies. He was the featured zydeco dancer in *Passion Fish,* director John Sayles's Oscar-nominated film set in South Louisiana. Joe appeared midway through the movie, in an evocative scene shot at Slim's Y-Ki-Ki. John Delafose and the Eunice Playboys, with Geno at the drums, were on the bandstand. And the man at center stage, in the black cowboy hat and facial hair, was Joe Potier. The moment exactly captures the sound and feel of a Creole dance club.

A few years later, in 1997, Joe appeared in *Eve's Bayou,* the Samuel Jackson film. "They were looking for dancers in New Orleans," Potier recalled, "and they went to a place called the Rock 'n' Bowl, where I happened to be dancing. So I was dancing like I usually dance, and as I was dancing, somebody tapped me on my shoulder. I said, 'What's a man doing tapping me on my shoulder while I'm dancing?' And as I was down dancing on the floor and stuff, this guy pulls out a contract. He said, 'You're the man. We got to have you in our movie.'"

Wildman appeared, in a much restrained form, in the film's opening scene, zydeco dancing at a house party. "They wouldn't let me do my moves," he complained. "Samuel Jackson said he didn't want any dancer stealing his show."

Despite his fame and dance-floor skills, Joe Potier said he often lacked for dance partners. "A lot of the black women don't dance with me. They say I intimidate them, or I make them look bad, or I dance too fancy. So I get a lot of rejection, 50 percent or more. But I don't get rejected by the white girls at all, because they see how much I like to dance, and they say they enjoy the way I dance and the amount of energy I put into it.

"I get criticized for dancing with them," he added. "People say, 'You like to dance with them white girls,' and I tell them point-blank, the white girls come to dance. If I paid my money at the door, I'm going to dance with whoever."

The objections, Joe said, often came from Creole women, who believed that Potier, by dancing with white women, was encouraging other black men to do the same. "They think that the white dancers were trying to take the black men. One of my white friends from Chicago, who'd been coming to Slim's for years, said she went to the bathroom there, and some black girls told her, 'Hey, we don't like your dancing with our black men.' It's a form of jealousy more than anything."

Creole men have also complained about Joe Potier's behavior. "I got threatened by the men at Thibodeaux's once," Wildman said. "It was the first time I went there, and three black guys were sitting at the bar. There were lots of ladies in the club. So these guys came up, and they said, 'Man, what are you doing here? Aren't you the guy that be dancing on TV all the time on *Zydeco Extravaganza*? I said, 'Yeah.' They said, 'Well, you need to go back to Lafayette.' So I'm looking at these three, and I said, 'Man, look. I'm going to tell you one thing. Number one, you saw me on TV. Number two, I'm here to dance. Number three, I'm staying here because I paid my money at the door.' So they told me, 'Well, man, we don't think that's a good idea.' I said, 'Well, you all give me a reason why I should leave.' 'Because you came to steal our women,' they said. I said, 'Man, look. I'm going dancing.' So I started dancing with the women. After a few dances I went to get me a soda at the bar. They came back and said, 'Man, see what we're talking about? You got all our women.' I said, 'Man, first of all, I didn't come here to find no woman. I don't have *a* woman. I'm dancing with *all* the women. And if you all would get away from the bar and just drinking and looking, maybe you all would have those women, too.'"

Joe Potier and I chatted for nearly two hours that evening. When it was over, I told him I had heard that Club Spice, a Lafayette dance place, had a zydeco band on tap that night.

"L'il Pookie is playing," I said. "You want to go check it out? You can show me how you dance."

"Yeah, oh yeah," he said.

Club Spice was located in a scruffy section of Lafayette, not far from the place Diana Steele and I had stayed on my first trip to the city. The club's distinctive feature was a rotating crystal ball that hung from the ceiling. I had never seen one of those in a zydeco dance hall before.

There was a small crowd there, and L'il Pookie waited until nearly eleven o'clock to start the show. Joe said he'd heard that the young accordionist, whose real name was Jimmy Seraile Jr., was suffering from the flu. But once L'il Pookie got going, his music sounded fine. Wildman roused up a dance partner and stepped out onto the floor.

Joe Potier was, by his own admission, subdued on the dance floor that night, eschewing his celebrated ground moves. It was late, he said, and he was tired.

But Wildman, even self-contained, was the most fluid, loosest zydeco dancer I had ever seen. I took notes while I watched him perform:

"Each limb of his body moves with amazing fluency. He seamlessly shifts from style to style. At one moment his legs dip to the ground with his hands on his hips like a Russian cossack. At another point he makes like a belly dancer. His body mostly undulates, as if seized by a wave that begins at his head and rolls down to his toes. He uses every joint in his torso: arching and bending with wonderful gestures that punctuate the music. While shining in the open position, his partner seems incidental, an anchor to his showmanship. When he closes back up, he overtakes her, lifts her lightly aloft, and moves her as he desires."

While I was watching Wildman, a Creole woman approached and pulled me onto the dance floor. She was middle-aged and very thin. She carried a beer in one hand and determination in the other. The lady was drunk, although I didn't pick up on her inebriation until midway through the dance, when the contents of her beer can spilled all over the floor. When the music ended, the woman hugged me and pulled me close, even as I tried to push her away.

She whispered in my ear, "I like you." Her speech was slurred.

Her assault brought to mind an incident I had suffered at Tornado Alley, several years before. An intoxicated lady, who was white, had somehow become my zydeco partner. She took to kissing me on the neck in the middle of our dance. I was appalled, and shoved her aside when she tried to linger on.

I chose more cordial tactics with my Club Spice Creole partner, not wanting to offend. I thanked the woman for the dance and tried, again, to walk away. She grabbed my arm, whirled me around, and angrily shouted: "ARE YOU WALKING AWAY FROM ME?"

"Thanks for the dance," I said, retreating from the dance floor, where Wildman was still holding forth, and where, I vowed, I would never again dance with a woman, whatever her race, who coddled herself in beer.

13
The Last Dance

It really was a shame that Coco Glass, my Cajun and zydeco teacher and friend, had never danced with Wildman. And had never visited Richard's Club or the Offshore Lounge or Slim's Y-Ki-Ki. I always believed that if she had gone to the source of the dance she enjoyed so much, she wouldn't have given it all up, as if it had never been there at all, just for the sake of a man. The loss would have seemed too dear.

The relationship at issue was, I suppose, worth the risk, for it certainly held promise. And the guy, whom I'd met, was actually quite nice, for a fellow who didn't like to dance. But in the end, things collapsed, another case of love gone wrong. And by the time the romance had played itself out, Coco Glass had changed too much to go back to the dance floor.

Her spirits, once buoyed by the push of an accordion and the scrape of a rubboard, had faltered, so much so that I wondered whether depression might have settled in. Her energy, once inexhaustible, had noticeably waned. Her spark and smile and appetite for fun, which had pulled me through my crisis with panic disorder, had lost their edge, or vanished altogether. All she did was work and sleep. She reminded me of me. Or the me I once was before I had made her acquaintance.

"Why did you stop dancing?" I asked her many, many months later, when the sting of the experience had eased. It was Thanksgiving time, and Coco had come for a visit. We hadn't seen each other for several years, and we passed a long weekend reminiscing, and sharing thoughts about social dance.

She responded to my question after a long silence. She chose her words with care.

"Because I developed other interests in my life that took up some of the time and space once filled by dancing," she said. "To be precise, a very important relationship with a nondancer.

"He had initially expressed a desire to learn how to dance," she recalled. "He loved the music, and he went to Louisiana on his honeymoon with his first wife. So I entered the relationship expecting to have the opportunity to introduce him to the dance community and to teach him how to dance. But after we went to several dances, it was clear he was uncomfortable. He was intimidated by all the experienced dancers. He was keeping company with the teacher, yet he didn't know how to dance. He felt that made him look bad, and he told me exactly that.

"I tried to teach him one-on-one, but he didn't seem to be interested," Coco explained. "But at that point the relationship seemed to have a lot of potential, more than with anybody I'd run across in a long time. And that was important to pursue. So basically, having to choose between him and dancing, I chose him.

"So I slowly but surely quit going to dances altogether. And I felt a little bit funny about that. I missed it because it had been such a huge part of my life. It was part of my regular routine. I was very aware when I gave it up of the impact it had on me.

"I lost contact with a social community that I had been part of and that had enriched me. I lost that regular outlet of exercise. I gained weight. I got out of shape. I had less energy. I had back trouble. Emotionally, I did not have the stress outlet that I'd had before, the thing that keeps you balanced and gives you a way, as I used to say, 'to get your yayas out' and to blow off steam. The frequency of my migraine headaches increased."

"Do you blame him for taking you away from the dance floor?" I asked.

"No, " she said. "Not really. I don't want to come off as sounding bitter. I thought he was the one I was looking for, and I thought he was interested in the same social activities as I was. It was wonderful. It was perfect. What a disappointment that it didn't work out."

After the relationship ended, Coco left the country. She moved to Caracas, Venezuela, where she had once lived, and where she had managed to find a job. "There is social dancing there," she said. "Salsa and merengue. But the culture is different, and a lady can't just show up on her own without a partner. I didn't have anyone to go with."

She later returned to the United States, but still stayed away from the dance floor. "I'm not sure why," she said, her uncertainty genuine. "Lack of motivation. Laziness. Loss of interest. Being out of shape. All those things.

"I am disconnected to the dance floor now, and it's hard to reach out and reconnect," she said. "Since I let go I've become an outsider. If I go out dancing I might feel like a beginner again, and maybe the sense of self-confidence I once had won't be there, and that discomforts me.

"I still think of myself as a dancer," Coco said, "at least when I talk to people who don't know me well. But when anybody asks me when I last went dancing, it's certainly not in the present tense.

"I can get the dance floor back," she insisted. "But I won't have the same place on it that I used to. And that's a shame."

Coco stopped speaking, drew a breath, and released a long, wistful sigh. It was time for a pause in our conversation.

We didn't talk about dance again until the weekend had nearly come to an end. We knew each other well enough to find pleasure in other less complicated things. We rented a film, *Primary Colors,* and talked about President Clinton. We walked in the park. We ate. A lot. Thanksgiving turkey and oven-baked yams. Sesame bagels with cream cheese and lox. Chocolate cake and nonfat frozen yogurt, the salves that soothe the soul.

She told me about her new career, which had brought her, at least temporarily, first to Minnesota, then back to her parents in Birmingham, the city she grew up in. She was living in her old house, she said, with her Alabama memories, and she had found a great deal of comfort in that. Sometimes it's good to cling to the past, she observed, for it helps to define a course for the future.

On our last evening together, as we slouched in some sofas over cups of chamomile tea, the conversation returned to the dance floor:

CoCo: What I miss most about dancing is the
    fun. The joy it used to bring to me.
ME: What do you think it is about dancing
    that makes it so much fun?
CoCo: It has to do with the interaction between
    two people, I think. You get to meet someone
    and focus your attention on them and try to
    function as a team. And the more successful
    you are at that, the more fun I think it is.
    And when it works, you just forget about
    everything else, you know? You become
    part of the music and the movement. You're
    just there, swallowed up in the moment.
    And then you fill the dance floor with this
    phenomenon. You fill it with lots of couples
    all doing the same thing, each one connected
    to the other, each one connected to the band,

and the band connecting the whole room. It is joyful. It's a feeling that's not replicated in any other setting.

ME: You know, I once asked Roy Carrier, the zydeco bandleader, about that connection you're talking about, between the dancers and the band. I asked him how he, as a lead performer, reacts to the dancers in front of him. Roy said something that surprised me. He said that dancers give him courage. And at first I didn't quite understand what he meant. And he talked about how difficult it was for him to stand onstage in front of a group of people who were depending on him to entertain them and to make them happy. And he said he was able to do it, night after night, only because of the dancers. He looked out into the crowd and fed off of that joyfulness you spoke of. It's the joyfulness that made him strong and gave him the courage to perform. And I realized that Roy had put his finger on it. That he had found in the dance hall a connection to humanity that empowers every man and woman in the room.

COCO: Is that what helped you to recover? That connection to humanity?

ME: Yeah. It absolutely gave me the courage to fight my panic disorder. In dancing the connection is quite literal—you're embracing other human beings, and sharing a joyful moment with them, and that is potent medicine. As time went on I felt that dancing thoroughly released the grip of the disease. But I'm wondering, in hindsight, if that was a process that you could observe.

Coco: I saw your anxiety, but, to be honest, I attributed that to shyness, not to something more serious, at least until you told me what was going on. And I saw someone who was terribly self-conscious on the dance floor. And most of all, I saw that for you there was an issue of perfection. You wanted to be good before you ever stepped out on the dance floor.

Me: You noticed.

Coco: Oh, yeah. Absolutely.

Me: Perfection was the thing that did me in. I was so obsessed with getting things right that I never learned how to have a good time.

Coco: Well, eventually you did. I saw you become a happier person. You stopped thinking so hard about everything you did. You became more confident and comfortable, less stiff and less wooden. Dancing gave you joy. And something besides your work to talk about. And you made new friends and became part of a community.

Me: Yeah, meeting new people was really important. Especially women. That's the great thing about social dancing when you're single and looking around. The activity itself is really fun. But beyond that, the possibility of meeting someone is always on the margins, it's always out there looming. It creates an edge that made the dances all the more interesting because of their unpredictability. You never knew what the next dance would bring.

Coco: Or who.

I met Eriko in Tornado Alley, the Wheaton, Maryland, nightclub, at a zydeco event in November 1994. They called her the "Asian Cajun," for she was born in Japan and loved Louisiana music. "The sound is unconditionally uplifting," she said. And so, said anyone who had danced with her, was Eriko.

She knew how to Cajun and zydeco extraordinarily well, so naturally and with so much flair that once, at Richard's Club in rural Lawtell, a perplexed Creole man who had danced with her shook his disbelieving head and said: "Where you from? Baton Rouge?" In fact she was from Kobe, the Japanese seaport, and had come to the States for graduate study, and then for a job as a journalist in Washington, D.C. She picked up Louisiana dancing at the local D.C. clubs.

Eriko had chocolate-brown eyes that twinkled with whimsy whenever she grinned, and a mane of long black hair that flowed down her back like a waterfall.

Samurai blood ran through her veins, which steeled her body and fortified her spirit. She was hard not to notice: a presence on the dance floor.

We danced together once that evening, but barely even spoke.

I didn't see Eriko again until the end of December, when we both joined a small group of people who went to South Louisiana to celebrate the new year. I was seriously attracted to her, and had hoped she would be part of the trip.

On the night before New Year's Eve, the group went to Thibodeaux's, a lovely, old two-story zydeco dance hall that sat on the cusp of Interstate 10 in Lake Charles. The house was thick with ambiance. Geno Delafose's band was onstage, pumped and sounding great, its pulse especially strong. Geno wore a cowboy hat and was singing in French with a honey-sweet tenor that went down like bread pudding. The hall itself was festooned on all sides in crepe paper and Christmas lights. Ladies in their Sunday best dished out bowls of potluck etouffeé. Gentlemen in hats and ties drank one-dollar Budweisers and diet Cokes.

The dance floor was large and spacious.

It was an intoxicating scene.

I asked Eriko to zydeco. And we did. One dance. A second. A third and a fourth, all in a row.

"I really like dancing with you," I told her afterward.

Eriko blushed for a moment, then beamed with appreciation. "You do?" she said. "Thanks. You're fun to dance with, too."

With Eriko something was palpably different. We danced with an inexplicable ease, even though we had barely danced before. When we twirled to the music we twirled with such speed that I thought we might go airborne; yet the revolutions, in my mind at least, were processed in slow motion, as if better to capture and savor the experience. And then there was that smile of hers, which never once diminished, regardless of the flow of dance. It just glowed, in an uncomplicated way. By the end of the night, when we went our separate ways, I had been done in. I resolved then and there to court her.

We were married a year later, on New Year's Day, on the back porch of an old Creole cottage on the banks of Bayou Teche in Breaux Bridge, Louisiana.

Our dance friends were there at our wedding, a dozen or so from Washington, and a few more from Louisiana. Before we exchanged vows, as we stood outdoors in a winter sun, a Cajun acquaintance named Dicky Breaux, who was hosting the gathering, announced that he wanted to read a poem. It was called "Bayou Epiphany," and Dicky had asked a New Orleans poet, Brod Bagert, to write it especially for the occasion:

> *Eriko and Robert were wed this New Year's Day.*
> *On the batteur of Bayou Teche,*
> *In a Caribbean Creole cottage,*
> *Wreathed by a dozen friends,*
> *They stood hand in hand,*
> *Breathed in cool evening air,*
> *Breathed out warm promises*
> *and waltzed into the moment of beginning.*

Beneath their feet
One hundred year old cypress boards held firm.
A hundred yards away the bayou flowed
As it has for a hundred thousand years.
Yet here—

This New Year's Day—
When Eriko and Robert gave promises,
As men and women often do,
The earth sang the song of love . . .
And the melody was new.

After the judge pronounced us husband and wife, and after we kissed, Dicky raised his eyes toward the heavens and whooped out *"Aiyee!"* the traditional Cajun holler. Thus blessed, we turned on some music, and Eriko and I consummated our marriage with an old Cajun waltz.

I think often of Dicky's gesture, of his cheery and heartfelt and piercing cry. He couldn't have known its effect on me: that the cry, like an exorcist's incantation, would scatter away from the cellar of my mind the un-settling remainders, the niggling fragments, of the panic disorder that had once controlled my life; and that the groom, thus fully cleansed, would be able to enter his marriage joyful and whole, calm and unencumbered.

Years later, Eriko and I are still dancing. We do Cajun and zydeco and occasionally some ballroom and swing. We dance with our son, Ariel, and with Katrina, his younger sister. The dancing still heals and nour-ishes, though, for me, the need and the urgency have diminished with time. I dance now because I want to, not because I have to. I dance for the fun, which I have learned to embrace. I dance for the exercise and the chance to make friends. I dance for my wife, who still smiles when we spin, and remains my very best partner. I still take dancing seriously, I suppose, for I'll always be a scholarly fellow. And out on the dance floor, I try, still, to perform with some sense of perfection. But per-fection, for me now, has an easy gait, and steps, almost always, in time with the music.

Postscript

Millions of Americans suffer from anxiety and related disorders. One expert has estimated that "up to 10% of the population experience sporadic panic attacks."[1] A study published by the National Institutes of Health says panic disorder "will afflict at least 1 out of every 75 people in this country and worldwide during their lifetime."[2]

Antianxiety drugs and psychotherapy, often in combination, can help most panic disorder sufferers to feel better. For each patient, the journey of recovery almost certainly traverses its own unique ground, shaped by the distinctive experiences and personality of the individual involved. For me, social dancing, and Cajun and zydeco dancing in particular, was transforming. The question is: Why? What was it about the dance floor that enabled me to overcome panic disorder?

I posed the question to Dr. Steven Gilbert. "My best guess," he said, "is that it is some combination of

1. M. Katherine Shear, "What's New in Medicine: Anxiety Disorders," in WebMD Scientific American Medicine, posted on Medscape Today, August 8, 2003. URL: www.medscape.com/viewarticle/459283

2. See "Panic Disorder: Consensus Statement," NIH/National Institute of Mental Health Consensus Development Conference, Sept. 25–27, 1991, 9.2, p. 3.

social and exercise therapy that is beneficial. We know that when people feel supported, when they have social supports, they seem to manage pain better. They seem to have somewhat better outcomes in cancer treatment and, in a particularly interesting study, had fewer complications during pregnancy and delivery." Dr. Gilbert did not know of any relevant studies regarding panic disorder, and my own research into the subject could not uncover any, either. But the socialization aspect of dancing—the sense of belonging to a dance community, of making the acquaintance of dozens of new friends—was an important element of my recovery. Coco Glass had it right when she told me that a family is a circle of friends who love you. On the dance floor, I found a family of friends who provided a support network and a kind of emotional sustenance I lacked in the earlier incarnation of my life. Their friendship surely made a difference.

As for exercise, it certainly is an element of social dancing, especially of zydeco, which can be extremely vigorous. One of my dance-floor companions once coined the term *zydaerobics* to describe the physical side of zydeco dance. Another likened a night of zydeco dancing to running a ten-kilometer race. Dr. Gilbert noted that aerobic exercise, "especially involving repetitive motion, is most likely to provide an antidepressant effect." A range of scientific studies, he said, has shown that to be the case. If aerobic exercise can help fend off depression, he surmised that it might play some role in fighting back panic disorder. Dancing certainly involves repetitive motion, and zydeco dancing, along with the Cajun jig, embraces that repetition, respectively, with quick side-to-side and up-and-down patterns.

My own view, however, is that it is the music, the high-beam force of the Cajun and zydeco accordion, which, when thrown into the mix of socialization and exercise, can blow away all semblance of anxiety. I am no scientist. But I do know that neuroscientists have shown that music can literally alter the brain and the emotions it produces.

Jaak Panksepp, a distinguished professor of psychobiology at Bowling Green State University, studies the impact of music on the brain. He says that there sits within the brain a still-to-be-defined mechanism that releases emotions when triggered by music. "We can easily make that assumption," Panksepp told me. "Everyone says that the main reason they listen to music is because it changes their emotions and moods, but how does that occur? Right now we're at a theoretical stage, where one can generate hypotheses, and the hypotheses are very straightforward because the auditory system and the emotional systems in the brain are very closely linked."

What that means, Panksepp said, is that "certain musical sounds and passages can have direct access to the brain's emotional systems, and the emotional systems in the brain are widely ramifying. So they will affect the tone of the whole nervous system, and that can have widespread consequences in terms of health consequences, mood consequences, cognitive consequences."

Add dance to the mix, and the consequences on mood are enhanced. Panksepp argues that music and dance are neurologically linked—partners, so to speak, on the dance floor of your mind. When music and dance work together, he says, the human brain has the capacity to express emotions in rhythmic body movements. It has always been that way.

"The ancestral relationship between movement and sound is probably fundamental to our nature," Panksepp said. "The impact of music on the brain systems that control bodily movement is profound."[3]

Panksepp has used an electroencephalogram, a scanning device that measures electrical activity in the brain, to look at the effect listening to music can have on the gray matter inside our heads. Interestingly, he found "that happy music tends to produce a more relaxed brain, whereas sad music tends to produce a more aroused brain. And for many people this seems paradoxical. They think about happy music as sort of getting more excited. But when you look at the EEG it appears to be more relaxed."

Happy music produces a more relaxed brain. A bit of neuroscientific evidence, perhaps, that may help to explain why Cajun and zydeco music and dance loosened the hold that anxiety once had on me.

3. Jaak Panksepp and Günther Bernatzky, "Emotional Sounds and the Brain: The Neuro-affective Foundations of Musical Appreciation," *Behavioral Processes* 60 (2002): 133–55, quote on p. 140.

Discography

Three of the great zydeco musicians who appear in this memoir have died since the events of the book took place: John Delafose passed away in 1994 at age fifty-five; Beau Jocque died in 1999 at age forty-five; and Boozoo Chavis died in 2001 at age seventy. Their recordings are still on the market. Of the songs mentioned in this memoir, by these artists and others, the following are commercially available. They are listed in the order they appear in the book:

"Down at the Twist and Shout," on Mary Chapin Carpenter's album *Shooting Straight in the Dark* (Sony, 1990)

"Tuxedo Junction," on *The Essential Glenn Miller* (RCA, 1995)

"Coeur des Cajuns," on Bruce Daigrepont's album *Coeur des Cajuns* (Rounder, 1989)

"Bosco Stomp," performed by Filé, on the album *La Musique Chez Mulate's* (Swallow, 1994)

"O yaie, bébé" is from the song "Two-step à Will Bolfa," on Beausoleil's album *Live! From the Left Coast* (Rounder, 1989)

"Jolie Blonde," performed by Dewey Balfa, can be heard on the album *La Musique Chez Mulate's* (Swallow, 1994)

"Watch that Dog" and "Go Back Where You Been," on
    John Delafose with Geno Delafose, *Pere et Garçon Zy-
    deco* (Rounder, 1992)
"Dance All Night," on Boozoo Chavis's album *Johnnie Billy
    Goat* (Rounder, 2000)
"Paper in My Shoe," "Dog Hill," "Leona Had a Party," and
    "Motor Dude Special" are all on Boozoo Chavis's *Zydeco
    Trail Ride* (Maison de Soul, 1990)
"Zydeco Extravaganza," on the Zydeco Force album *Shaggy
    Dog Two-Step* (Maison de Soul, 1992)
"Give Him Cornbread," on Beau Jocque's *Beau Jocque Boo-
    gie* (Rounder, 1993)

My favorite albums by Cajun and zydeco artists mentioned
in this memoir:

Amédé Ardoin: *The Roots of Zydeco* (Arhoolie, 1995)
Beausoleil: *Live! From the Left Coast* (Rounder, 1989)
Beau Jocque and the Zydeco Hi-Rollers:
    Beau Jocque Boogie (Rounder, 1993)
    Git It, Beau Jocque (Rounder, 1995)
Boozoo Chavis and the Majic Sounds:
    Live! At the Habibi Tample (Rounder, 1994)
    Boozoo, That's Who! (Rounder, 1993)
    Zydeco Homebrew (Maison de Soul, 1992)
Roy Carrier and the Night Rockers:
    Zydeco Strokin' (Paula Records, 1995)
    Nasty Girls (Right on Rhythm, 1996)
Clifton Chenier: *Bon Ton Roulet!* (Arhoolie, 1990)
Geno Delafose: *French Rockin' Boogie* (Rounder, 1994)
Steve Riley and the Mamou Playboys: *La Toussaint*
    (Rounder, 1995)
Zydeco Force: *Shaggy Dog Two-Step* (Maison de Soul, 1992)

Coco Glass's five favorite Cajun albums (with an assist from
Chris Trahan):

Bruce Daigrepont:
  Coeur des Cajuns (Rounder, 1989)
  Stir Up the Roux (Rounder, 1987)
  Petit Cadeu (Rounder, 1994)
Steve Riley and the Mamou Playboys: *Steve Riley and the
  Mamou Playboys* (Rounder, 1990)
Filé: *Live at Mulate's* (Flying Fish, 1985)

Ben Pagac's five favorite zydeco albums (with his comments):

Boozoo Chavis, *Zydeco Trail Ride* (Maison de Soul, 1990).
  "What more could you ask for—one disk, twenty-one
  songs, all approximately three minutes long. That means
  twenty-one different dance partners with energy to
  spare! Boozoo once said, 'I can play one hundred songs
  in one hour—and you know I play them right!'"
Zydeco Force, *Shaggy Dog Two-Step* (Maison de Soul, 1992).
  "The *White Album* of Zydeco. The song 'Zydeco
  Extravaganza' single-handedly conjures up the excitement of seeing a line of parked cars stretched out along
  the shoulder of Route 190 and ending at a plain, wooden
  building with a yellow-light sign out front."
J. Paul Jr. and the Zydeco Newbreeds, *Another Level* (World
  Wide Music, 1999). "The contemporary Houston zy-
  deco dance scene finds a powerful ambassador."
Keith Frank & the Soileau Zydeco Band, *Live at Slim's Y-Ki-
  Ki* (Shanachie, 1999). "The recording of a live zydeco
  dance-hall performance has never sounded so good . . .
  until now."
Brian Jack & the Zydeco Gamblers, *Give Me Some Room*
  (BJZG, 2000). "Another Houston talent. The songs
  'Mudfish,' 'Shake & Bake,' and 'Step Back, Give Me
  Some Room' (a Roy Carrier cover) vary widely in tem-
  pos yet are all foot-grabbing."